Return to the
SOURCE

God's Design for Nutrition

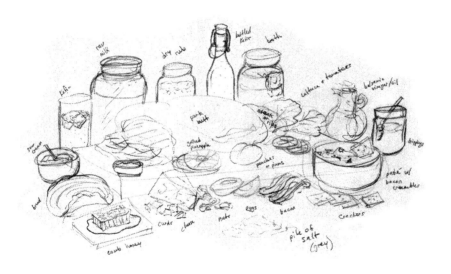

KELLY HAMBELTON

WESTBOW
PRESS®
A DIVISION OF THOMAS NELSON
& ZONDERVAN

This book is a work of non-fiction. Unless otherwise noted, the author
and the publisher make no explicit guarantees as to the accuracy of
the information contained in this book and in some cases, names of
people and places have been altered to protect their privacy.

All Scripture quotations, unless otherwise indicated, are taken from the Holy
Bible, New International Version®, NIV®. Copyright ©1973, 1978, 1984, 2011
by Biblica, Inc.™ Used by permission of Zondervan. All rights reserved worldwide.
www.zondervan.com The "NIV" and "New International Version" are trademarks
registered in the United States Patent and Trademark Office by Biblica, Inc.™

Scripture taken from the King James Version of the Bible.

WestBow Press books may be ordered through booksellers or by contacting:

WestBow Press
A Division of Thomas Nelson & Zondervan
1663 Liberty Drive
Bloomington, IN 47403
www.westbowpress.com
1 (866) 928-1240

Because of the dynamic nature of the Internet, any web addresses or
links contained in this book may have changed since publication and
may no longer be valid. The views expressed in this work are solely those
of the author and do not necessarily reflect the views of the publisher,
and the publisher hereby disclaims any responsibility for them.

Any people depicted in stock imagery provided by Getty Images are
models, and such images are being used for illustrative purposes only.
Certain stock imagery © Getty Images.

ISBN: 978-1-9736-3108-8 (sc)
ISBN: 978-1-9736-3109-5 (hc)
ISBN: 978-1-9736-3107-1 (e)

Library of Congress Control Number: 2018906999

Print information available on the last page.

WestBow Press rev. date: 8/30/2018

"My people are destroyed from lack
of knowledge." Hosea 4:6a

"O my people, hear my teachings; listen to the words
of my mouth. I will open my mouth in parables, I will
utter hidden things, things from of old – what we have
heard and known, what our fathers have told us. We will
not hide them from our children; we will tell the next
generation the praiseworthy deeds of the LORD, his
power, and the wonders he has done." Psalm 78:1-4

"Then we will no longer be infants, tossed back and forth
by the waves, by every wind of teaching and by the cunning
and craftiness of men in their deceitful scheming. Instead,
speaking the truth in love, we will in all things grow up into
him who is the Head, that is, Christ." Ephesians 4:14-15

NIV Study Bible

For all those whose stories I've listened to as they told of their family and children who struggle with ADHD, allergies, asthma, and diabetes.

For all of those whose tear-filled discussions describing their painful struggle with obesity, stomach surgeries, sickly children, and ill family members that touched me so deeply.

For those who have asked me countless questions about food and where to start making changes to their diets.

For those who have struggled with food allergies, asthma, and eczema.

For my husband who bravely tasted many strange foods and put up with endless unlabeled jars, pickles, and fermented bubbly "food" in our kitchen. I applaud his courage and thank him for his support for me in writing this book and taking this journey with me. I could not have done this without him.

For my Lord and Savior, who answered my prayers when I sat tearfully looking at a string of bottles of pills for headaches, allergies, colds and asked, "Lord, what do I do? There has to be a better way." Funny, I always thought the Lord would answer my prayers by helping me find a book about medicine, or help me take an online class about drugs and medicine, or perhaps even help me befriend a nurse who could answer my questions. What I ended up learning was a complete surprise.

Acknowledgment and Thanks

Thank you, Lord, for taking me on this journey. I love the twists and turns, surprises and challenges that keep me pressing forward. Thank you for giving me the chance to learn all the things I have learned about food so far, and the things I will learn in the future. Thank you for giving my husband and me the dream of teaching this material to others, to lead them to you.

Thank you, my husband, for believing and trusting God enough to dive wholeheartedly into this journey. You trusted God enough to wander with me into uncharted territory and try new things. You trusted enough to pack up our family, sell our home and move onto a small farm and get your hands dirty, even though neither of us had ever lived on a farm. Thank you for encouraging me to write this book and giving me the courage to continue when I wanted to quit.

Thank you, my daughters, for helping me with photography and setting up photos of spices and different foods.

Thank you to my friends who encouraged me to write this book, proofread the text, tested recipes, and invested in its publication. Thank you Carli Phillips, Joe LaCognata, and Karen Bhaggan for giving up your precious time to read and proofread this text.

Thank you to all of those who have come before me and paved the way for me to learn and understand the material written in this book. Thank you to the Weston Price Foundation for teaching others about traditional foods. Thank you to Joel Salatin and all those at Polyface Farm for giving my husband and me the inspiration to leave the city and begin raising our own food. Thank you to Dr. Natasha Campbell-McBride for all of her research about natural foods that heal the gut. Her book, Gut and Psychology Syndrome, was instrumental in helping our family heal many of the gut problems that we used to have. I would also like to thank Sue Becker for introducing our family to home-ground wheat, an essential step in our family's healing journey. Thank you also to Sally Fallon Morell for writing Nourishing Traditions, the first book I read that opened my eyes to a different way of eating and redefined healthy food. Thank you, also, to Sonlight homeschool curriculum for carrying Nourishing Traditions as their textbook on health, where I first saw and purchased Nourishing Traditions.

How to Use This Book

This book is laid out in three main sections – God's Word, God's Design, and Understanding Fresh Food. Please read the first two sections, God's Word and God's Design, before continuing on to the cooking instruction in Understanding Fresh Food. It is vitally important that you understand the material in the first two sections so that you know how to obtain ingredients to make the items in section three. The third section, Understanding Fresh Food, is meant to be used as a manual for cooking and preparing delicious food for your family. It can be used as a reference or simply read through to spark ideas and your cooking imagination. Enjoy!

Please know I humbly present these thoughts and ideas from personal experience and some very brilliant people that I have been fortunate to come across in my personal search for health. I do not claim to be a physician, dietician, or nutritionist. I encourage everyone to speak with their doctor and find what works best for your family.

Contents

Introduction

I've written this book to help families make sense of the good and bad information deluge we are all experiencing. Families feel lost and confused when shopping the supermarket aisles. There's a sinking feeling I get when someone asks me "I want to start making some changes to my diet, but where should I begin?" I've tried giving people a list of websites to explore or a book to begin reading, but I haven't found a resource yet that combines "what to eat" with "where your food comes from" and "why you shouldn't believe that advertising." Families need easy-to-apply answers. Most research does not respect God's design of our world. God's design is not reflected in the medical reviews that tell us to limit our salt or reduce our saturated fat intake. I honestly don't think we can make changes to our diet and succeed without some education about what is going on in our food system.

My goal for this book is to clarify God's definition of nutrition versus American ideals and marketing. I want to clearly define God's design and help you use that as a benchmark for comparing "research," setting some boundaries on what we should and should not accept as truth. I also want to create a path to good nutrition that is easy to follow. This book is designed to help home cooks put food on the table and nourish their families.

We will first discuss what God's Word says about food and

nutrition. God has set clear patterns and instructions that many families do not understand or respect today. We pay for it with our health.

We will also discuss God's design of our world. This is very important to understand so that we do not fall victim to the ever-changing trends and marketing of our food. For example, it has been concluded that the cholesterol naturally present in egg yolks is bad for us. Why, then, would God place an egg yolk sac next to every human developing embryo full of "deadly" cholesterol?[1,2] This conclusion goes against God's design. If eggs have been researched and it is concluded they are bad for us, then we need to ask ourselves, "Is this correct research?" and, if it is, then "What are we doing wrong to the eggs?" Or better yet, "Are we raising our animals in accordance with God's design for them?" This is what I mean by *Return to the Source*. We need to return to the Creator's design for our food, and this means going back to the source of our food; back to the grass, back to the field, back to the seed.

Then we will discuss how to cook using fresh food; delicious, juicy, tasty, fresh food! I love to cook and watch people come wandering in from other rooms of the house, noses held high sniffing the air, asking, "Hey, what are you cooking?" God designed our food to be fun, beautiful, tasty, and nutritious all at the same time. May this book be an inspiration for you. But first, we need to know some things about how our food is grown and marketed in our food system.

Isaiah 46:4 NIV

> *"Even to your old age and gray hairs I am He, I am He who will sustain you. I have made you and I will carry you; I will sustain you and I will rescue you."*

BREAKING THE FOOD CHAINS

It's about freedom. God wants to free His people from the onslaught of bad information, a corrupt food and medicine paradigm, and outrageous weight loss ideals. All of this is bondage. God's people are in food bondage. We rely on "research" to tell us what we should be eating and how we should nourish our bodies, but we have forgotten that God has given us everything we need, including instruction on how we should nourish ourselves. Truth is freedom, and God wants us to know the truth. He designed this world for us, including all of our food, so that we could know Him and know His love for us. Why on earth would God create animal meat lined with delicious fat if animal fat was bad for us? Why would He design cream to rise to the top of milk and create milk so that it makes butter, cheese, yogurt, kefir, and sour cream if He did not want us to enjoy it? I've heard people say, "Everything that tastes good is bad for me." I want to challenge that idea.

We've been led to believe that animal fats are bad for us and that we should look to the USDA and FDA to set guidelines for us as to what we should eat and how much. We even have handy guidelines like "My Plate"[3] that tell us what proportions of vegetables and meat to eat. These are laughable, however, because they do not discriminate between a fast food hamburger and a homemade hamburger made from local, grass-fed beef raised in humane and healthy conditions. One could make you very sick and the other is nourishing, following God's design. Many fast food hamburgers are made from CAFO (Concentrated Animal Feeding Operation) beef from feedlot cows raised in disgusting conditions with little or no grass, sometimes standing several feet deep in their own manure.[4] Local beef is raised by small farmers that take pride in raising healthy animals, out in their own fields in the clean air and sunshine. The meat, fat, bones, milk, and organs of these animals are fully nourishing and will help maintain a healthy body weight and normal blood cholesterol. Our family has lost weight and lowered our cholesterol by switching to local, fresh food. My husband no longer takes Prilosec for acid reflux and we stopped catching most colds. God's design for food works.

God is smarter than us. We have taken the foods He designed to nourish us and have processed them until they no longer resemble what He created. Is a box of fruit juice really equal to two servings of fruit? Are yogurt covered raisins really a great source of calcium? The dark side of convenient foods is that we don't understand how our bodies operate and we do much damage to ourselves by assuming that processed foods are equal to fresh, homemade foods. There are trillions of microscopic good bacteria living in our guts.[5] These good bacteria and enzymes break down our food and pull nutrition from the food we eat. Our bodies can only make a portion of the bacteria and enzymes we need to digest our food. The rest need to come from our food. Did you catch that? We need to eat a certain amount of *living* foods, foods that are alive. High-heat processing kills these nourishing bacteria and enzymes.

Let me give you an example. God created milk as a living food. It is full of enzymes and beneficial microflora. Lactose is a milk sugar, naturally occurring in all milk. Lactase is the enzyme needed to breakdown the milk sugar, lactose. Most people's bodies can make enough lactase to digest milk, but some cannot. When milk is pasteurized these lactase enzymes are destroyed leaving the body with the hard work of breaking down the lactose sugar all by itself. So this poses a question: do people who are lactose intolerant truly have a sensitivity to lactose or do they need to drink fresh, unpasteurized milk with all the included lactase enzymes in order to be able to digest the milk? There are many lactose-intolerant people who have switched to fresh, local, unpasteurized milk and have had great results; not all, but many. And this is only one example of how we are destroying our health with convenient, processed foods.

There are many more examples of how we are ruining our own food. The result is poor health, reliance on medicine to get through the day and much, much frustration.

This combination of lack of living foods and blindly accepting any food guidelines takes a dark twist when you take a closer look at the where the money goes. In the United States, Congress is responsible for passing a multibillion-dollar farm bill. Included are the guidelines for governing where taxpayer dollars go for subsidizing the food industry. Certain foods are subsidized by the government, causing subsidized foods to be artificially lower than the real cost of that food. Doesn't this provide food for the poor? Yes... but what kind of food? Low quality, cheap, processed foods to be exact. The farm bill was originally formed during the Great Depression to help feed the poor, but over time, food industry interests have clouded the purpose of the bill. Corn is one of the foods subsidized by our tax dollars. High fructose corn syrup is subsidized by our tax dollars, which helps explain why soda is less than a dollar for a two-liter. The very system designed to create food for the poor is making them sick by flooding the market with cheap junk food. Small farmers trying to produce fresh foods have a hard time competing with the food on supermarket shelves. We would be far better off to eliminate food subsidies and level the playing field so small farmers can compete and flood the market with local, fresh food. It would create hundreds of thousands of jobs. This is the driving momentum behind farmer's markets. They are popping up everywhere, and families are rejoicing at the availability of fresh, local food.

We're not done following the money yet. Next, take into account a bankrupting health care system that is also supported by our tax dollars. We are knee deep in cheap food as a nation. We subsidize corn syrup and then our health insurance pays for insulin pumps. This is what I call burning the wallet at both ends. Our tax dollars produce mountains of junk food, and then we bankrupt our nation caring for chronic health problems caused by all this processed food. None of this is God's design.

Finally, we have to look at the power of advertising and research. We have a profit-driven food system. The most money to be made is by producing items which are patentable. Drugs and medicine are patentable. Vitamins are not. Genetically modified foods (GMOs) and seeds are patentable. Fresh, local food is not. Genetically modified foods cover much of the junk food produced in the United States. This is why many attempts to pass laws labeling GMOs in our food have failed. This is not to restrict GMOs; it is only to *label* them, so consumers can see that genetically modified foods are listed in the ingredients. The food industry has paid millions of dollars in defeating GMO labeling laws.[6] They are so powerful that many states have passed labeling laws, but those laws specify that unless two or more adjoining states pass similar laws their law does not go into effect.[7,8] Why would a state wait for other adjoining states to also pass the same law? Because they live in fear. The food industry has so much power that the states fear a massive lawsuit from the food industry. It would be difficult for a single state government to take on the entire food industry by itself.

The power of the food and biotechnology industry goes further than that. The biotechnology industry is responsible for producing GMO food and seeds. These seeds are patentable by government law, meaning that the company owns the genetic material, the DNA, in the seed. These seeds are bought by farmers on a contract basis. By buying the seeds, the farmers are subject to their contract. Some contracts specify that a farmer cannot save any seed from their crops. This means they have to buy the seed every year.[9] This flies in the face of God's design, who designed this world to produce seeds that multiply freely. Ever cut open a pumpkin and dig out all those seeds? Each and every seed can be planted to create a whole new pumpkin vine the following year. So, if you have one pumpkin, open it and save the hundred or so seeds, you can plant a hundred pumpkin vines the following year.

This is God's plan for free food. Yet, these farmers are limited by the contract with the biotechnology companies to not save any seed. It is a bondage for them as well. So why not simply buy seeds that are non-GMO? There aren't enough seeds being produced to supply the farmers even if they wanted to switch. Not all at once, anyway. But many farmers are making the switch away from GMO seeds and their efforts should be rewarded.

The power of the biotechnology industry is stronger than the food industry. Let me tell you about a trial that went all the way to the Supreme Court. OSGATA, the Organic Seed Growers and Trade Association, went to trial against Monsanto Corporation, the largest producer of GMO soy.[10] Why were they angry with Monsanto? They were fighting for the right of farmers to *not* be sued by Monsanto when GMO pollen from Monsanto soybeans in nearby fields blew into their fields and cross-pollinated their soybeans. You see, these farmers were being sued for having Monsanto soy DNA in their soy beans even though they had not purchased Monsanto soybeans or had any contract with them. Dozens of organic seed alliances, exchanges, and small farmers joined the lawsuit to be rid of the harassment from this biotechnology company. The result? The case was dismissed. It never went to full trial. You see, there is too much at stake for Monsanto to risk losing their GMO patents, and no court is ready to challenge the monstrous biotechnology industry just yet. This is the same biotech industry that the states fear in passing GMO labeling laws. In reality, GMO patents should never have been awarded in the first place because the biotechnology industry cannot control the wind blowing pollen into others' fields. How do you hold a patent on something that God designed to multiply freely?

> How do you hold a patent on something that God designed to multiply freely?

The power of the food industry also shows itself in farm regulation and licensing. Since the licensing and regulating are carried out by organizations designed to help the food industry, small farmers often lose when it comes to battling for the right to produce and sell their products. In another trial, a small farmer named Hershberger had to fight for the right to sell his farm's fresh, raw milk to members of his buying club.[11,12] In June 2010, Wisconsin Department of Agriculture appeared on his farm and searched the property. They locked up his refrigerators where the milk was being stored until further notice and poured blue dye into the bulk tank, ruining nearly 300 gallons of fresh milk. This is commonly known as a milk raid. There had been no complaints of illness or sickness caused by the milk. Regulators argued that he did not have a license to sell unpasteurized milk. Hershberger countered that he only provided food to buyers in a private buying club, therefore, not requiring him to have a license. These are the kind of battles that are appearing in courts between large food industry regulators and small organic farmers. What's worse, there was a gag order on the trial and no one was allowed to say the words "raw milk." This is a lot of trouble for a paperwork discrepancy. It's competition. Farmer's markets hold the largest threat to the food industry. Every dollar consumers spend on local food and farmer's markets is a vote against big food industry. Please visit the Farm to Consumer Legal Defense Fund website for updates on food laws and a state-by-state list of current food and small farmer court trials (www.farmtoconsumer.org). There are ways you can help by calling your local legislators and supporting pro-small-farmer legislation.

There are many people trapped in this mess. Legislators have the difficult job of trying to pass laws that enable small farmers to compete with the larger food industry without trampling on the rights of commercial food producers. Regulators have the equally difficult task of making sure that the public has access to safe, clean food. Even commercial farmers are trapped by their contracts with food producers. They receive very little, only a small fraction, of the money from the sale of the food they have worked so hard to produce. Most consumers feel lost and don't know what to believe. Making healthy food choices at the supermarket for their families is a daunting task.

However, the story is not over. God wants us to be free and live in knowledge and truth. The good news is that it is much easier (and tastier!) to follow God's design for nutrition. Fresh food – every animal, every plant, every spice and flavor has been given to us for food. He would rather us be dependent on Him, and His fresh food and creation, than to be in the current bondage we find ourselves in now. There is hope in the Lord.

> *"Behold, I will bring it health and cure, and I will cure them, and will reveal unto them the abundance of peace and truth." Jeremiah 33:6, KJV.*

Thinking about our Health

When it comes to thinking about our health there are two extremes. On one hand, we have non-Biblical research telling us that as long as we get our "nutrients" we will be healthy. This is called "nutrientism" and is a sort of idolizing of man's achievements. In my opinion, The Food Guide Pyramid and My Plate are a sad illustration of this mind set. Eat a certain amount of fruits, veggies and grains, no matter how they are processed or pasteurized, and you should be healthy. I laugh when I see futuristic movies where people eat one vitamin or some sort of green goo and we are supposed to believe that they have received all the nutrition they need for the day. God created us to be a part of this world. Let us not underestimate His wisdom.

At the other end of the two extremes is idolizing "Nature." We are not made perfect by eating all plants and healthy foods. There are no sacred foods or "superfoods" that make us miraculously healthy. It would be cruel for

God to put a mineral crucial to our health only in, let's say, seafood, where people living far away from the ocean could not reach it. Even iodine is found in many other foods besides seafood. He also would not put a nutrient vital to our health in tropical plants alone, for those who live in harsh, arctic environments would not be able to thrive. Be wary of health foods that claim to be the only source of a vital nutrient or miraculous healing potential. Only God can heal us.

In the middle of these two extremes is God's design. We are dependent on the microscopic life embedded in our foods and on His blessing of our foods. We are also dependent on His wisdom in the design of our world and need to respect His design if we are going to be successful.

IS IT WORTH THE EFFORT TO COOK FROM SCRATCH?

Okay, I admit it. It's a lot of work to cook from scratch. Let me give you a few reasons why it's worth the extra effort:

> I used to think that having that full, bloated feeling after eating a large meal was normal... *it's not normal*. When we eat fresh home-ground bread and meat with gravy, we don't feel bloated. We feel fine.

> I used to think that acid reflux after eating was normal... *it's not normal*. That only happens now after we have eaten out at a restaurant. We can eat battered and fried foods at home with no acid reflux. We use fresh ingredients as close to the source as we can purchase or make them.

I used to think that having sugar crashes and that feeling of being tired and completely weak was normal... *it's not normal.* I learned how to balance my blood sugar and how to eat sugar with protein and fat so it doesn't mess up my blood sugar. And unexpectedly, when we started eating less sugar in general, my insulin resistance healed. It healed! I can actually eat a small piece of candy on an empty stomach now without feeling sick. Not that I try to do that, but I've noticed just how much my body has corrected its sugar problems when I corrected my food.

I used to think that having monthly menstrual cramps, with lower backpain and upset stomach was normal... *it's not normal.* That only happens on months when I know I haven't eaten enough liver and organ meats. These organ meats contain loads of folate (the natural form of folic acid) and minerals. The folate prevents menstrual cramps and symptoms altogether.

I used to think that getting sick from antibiotics was normal... *it's not normal.* I know now that if I drink one cup of raw milk or kefir each day while on antibiotics, I can take antibiotics for an infection and not feel any negative symptoms from the antibiotics. Taking antibiotics does, however, weaken my system and allow more infections to develop, so I immediately begin building back up my immune system with healthy microflora as soon as I can.

I used to think my daughter's behavior, emotional state, and lack of focus on her schoolwork were

what we had to live with... *that's not normal.*
If I see her acting out, becoming emotional and
hyperactive, I immediately begin reviewing her
diet. What has she eaten in the last few days?
Birthday cake? Candy? Fast food? Way too many
potato chips? The starch and sugar encourage
opportunistic microflora to build in her gut and
throw her gut and immune system off balance.
These microflora also release toxins into her gut,
that then go straight into her bloodstream.[13] We
buckle down and get her back on completely
homemade foods and the symptoms go away.
No medicine needed.

Making food from scratch is a fun kind of work. You get to
come home to the smell of roasts in the crock pot. On weekends,
the house smells of fresh baked bread. Snacks and breakfast are
pretty easy; a piece of homemade toast with butter and a sliced
apple or a hard-boiled egg. It's not the chips and ice cream that
children beg for, but they'll get over it. We have homemade
blueberry jam in the fridge. Put some of that on your toast.
There are homemade apple muffins – made with real butter,
cane syrup, fresh-ground flour and eggs. Have one for a snack.
It's not as bad as you think. There's homemade ice cream,
cheeses and yogurt; leftover pot roast to pack for your lunch.
It's actually quite delicious.

Section One
GOD'S WORD

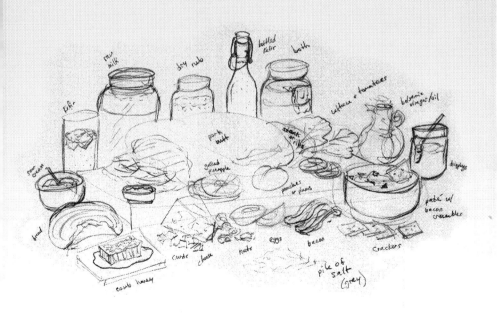

Kelly Hambelton

WISDOM FROM THE WRONG SOURCE

As Christ followers, we know that the Bible is the go-to reference for every aspect of our lives. If you want to know how to handle money or how to stay happily married, there are hundreds of Christian seminars and books to read about the topic. Parenting? Leadership? Again, loads of resources. Just browse a Christian book store for a few minutes and take a look at the multitude of books and DVDs. Why, then, do we go to secular government agencies for wisdom about food and diet?

The problem with trusting a secular agency to tell us what we should eat to be healthy is that they do not take into account God's Word and God's design of our world. When research told us in the 1980s that saturated fat was bad for us, everyone dumped their butter, trimmed the fat from their steaks, and began eating "healthy" vegetable oils. Thirty years later, these "healthy" vegetable oils are the suspect of many health problems, and butter is making a comeback. The same has been true of eggs: they are healthy, they are unhealthy... no, wait, they are healthy. But God and His design of our world does not change. Neither should our food.

> Why, then, do we go to secular government agencies for wisdom about food and diet?

These agencies are also subject to corruption. The USDA (United States Department of Agriculture) and the FDA (Food and Drug Administration) are monstrous agencies today. What started out with Abraham Lincoln in the mid-1800s as a small department to "diffuse among the people of the United States useful information... and to distribute among the people new and valuable seeds and plants" has swollen to employ thousands of people.[14] They control billions of dollars that dictate what our nation eats. Where there is that much power and money, corruption may surface. To complicate the situation, research and marketing are driven by sales and money-making potential. It seems there is a new "superfood" every week.

So how are God's people to know what to believe? We need to use God's Word and His design of our world as a measuring stick to compare the accuracy of all this information. We need to know what He says about food and nutrition. We need to understand His design of our world. It will keep us from falling prey to diet trends and marketing disguised as research. God has given us clear instruction about what to eat. If we understand His design of our food, we won't be confused by misleading research.

Here are three parameters to follow for sorting through our culture's "facts" about food:

Rule #1: Don't *ever* assume you know everything there is to know about God's creation. He and His design are far more complex than we can possibly imagine. It will keep us from making mistakes in our judgment, to always assume there is more to the picture than what we can see. Humility is required.

Rule #2: Does it agree with Scripture? When God called the Holy Land a "land of milk and honey," we can know that milk and honey are foods that God designed for us. If our culture's research says they are harmful, that ought to be a clue for us that we are doing something wrong to damage our food. We need to change what is damaging our food, not just remove it from our diet.

Rule #3: Does it agree with God's design of creation? If we have a good understanding of how God designed our food, it will keep us from falling victim to marketing and diet trends. Today, there are many diet trends that encourage people to avoid whole food groups. Why avoid all red meats? Why avoid carbs? Why avoid saturated fats? God designed them to be a natural part of a well-rounded diet. When research told us to remove saturated fat from our diets, it should have raised some serious questions. Saturated fat is in so many foods that God created. How do you remove it? It's in almost every meat and animal product. Removing saturated fats doesn't make sense. The same is true with carbs. They are a part of God's design. There are many recommendations for people to reduce their salt intake, but salt is a key ingredient for food preservation. Before refrigeration, food preservation was difficult without salt. Even the cattle in our fields have their own salt and mineral block to lick. Salt is necessary for life, so we need to ask ourselves, "Are we somehow ruining our salt by processing it?" Yes, even salt is processed. If research shows that a food is harmful for us, we need to ask ourselves, "Is this correct research," and if so, then, "What are we doing wrong?"

> Romans 12:2 "Do not conform any longer to the pattern of this world, but be transformed by the renewing of your mind. Then you will be able to test and approve what God's will is – his good, pleasing and perfect will."
>
> Ephesians 4:14-15 "Then we will no longer be infants, tossed back and forth by the waves, by every wind of teaching and by the cunning and craftiness of men in their deceitful scheming. Instead, speaking the truth in love, we will in all things grow up into him who is the Head, that is, Christ."

The Power of Repentance

Repentance - Greek: "metanoia", a *change* of mind.[15]

When I take a look at the world God created full of foods that He made to nourish us, several things come to mind. First, God cares for us. Look at the trouble He went through to make sure every continent has access to seas and grazing land. When I look at how beautiful and simple His design for food is, a genuine sorrow develops toward God because we, as a nation, have walked away from His design. Second, I begin to feel a distaste for the junk food man has created, and it pushes me forward to source real food. Third, it is humbling to realize how completely we depend on God for our health.

We need to repent for the decisions of people who came before us. Many of us were born into this mess of eating foods completely removed from their source. I grew up eating TV dinners and didn't know a thing about cattle or poultry, saving seeds, or harvesting fruit. As I began to learn about God's design for fresh, real food I began to value the hard work of farmers. I developed a love for learning. *I had a change of mind*. Please help me in praying for our nation in repentance. May we change our mind about our food.

DESIGNED FOR A SPECIAL PURPOSE

I think you will find this interesting. My daughters and I discovered this while studying their homeschool science book. Open your Bible to Genesis and look at the very beginning when God was creating the earth and all of its creatures. Take a look at the sixth day, the day God created land animals. Most people breeze over this part and say "God created animals and then God created man." Actually, God did not lump all "land animals" into the same category. Look at Genesis 1:24:

"And God said, 'Let the land produce living creatures according to their kinds: livestock, creatures that move along the ground, and wild animals, each according to its kind.' And it was so."

Did you catch that? God made an entire class of animals *from the beginning* that are designed to get along with humans: livestock. There are plenty of verses to back this up. Let's keep moving. Read verse 26:

"Then God said, 'Let us make man in our image, in our likeness, and let him rule over the fish of the sea and the birds of the air, over the livestock, over all the earth, and over all the creatures that move along the ground.'"

God gave man the assignment to rule over the fish and birds, livestock, earth (soil, ground), and over all the creatures that move along the ground. Notice that wild animals are not on that list. We were never made to rule over wild animals. Livestock, however, is designed to be under our rule. It's not an accident that horses and mules have strong backs that can carry us. It's not an accident that cows, goats, and sheep have a gentle nature and create large amounts of milk. They make milk that can be transformed into cream, butter and cheese. They were designed to be livestock. Now look at Genesis 2:19:

"Now the Lord God had formed out of the ground all the beasts of the field and all the birds of the air. He brought them to the man to see what he would name them; and whatever the man called each living creature, that was its name."

God brought only the beasts of the field and the birds. I find it funny that God didn't bring a string of lions, tigers, and bears and say, "Here, name these." He brought only the animals that man would have a close relationship with.

As for our food, God gives us our food in two stages. In Genesis 1:27-29, the Bible tells us this: "So God created man in his own image, in the image of God he created them; male and female he created them. God blessed them and said to them, 'Be fruitful and increase in number; fill the earth and subdue it. Rule over the fish of the sea and the birds of the air and over every creature that moves on the ground'. Then God said, 'I give you every seed-bearing plant on the face of the whole earth and every tree that has fruit with seed in it. They will be yours for food.'"

After the flood with Noah, God gives us the second stage. In Genesis 9:1-3, the Bible says, "Then God blessed Noah and his sons, saying to them, 'Be fruitful and increase in number and fill the earth. The fear and dread of you will fall upon all the beasts of the earth and all the birds of the air, upon every creature the moves along the ground, and upon all the fish of the sea; they are given into your hands. Everything that lives and moves will be food for you. Just as I gave you the green plants, I now give you everything.'"

My Bible has some interesting footnotes pertaining to the word "rule." The footnotes for Genesis 1:28 say this: "Humankind goes forth from the hands of the Creator under his divine benediction – flourishing, filling the earth with their kind, and exercising dominion over the other earthly creatures... Human culture, accordingly, is not anti-God (though fallen human beings often have turned their efforts into proud rebellion against God). Rather, it is the activity of those who bear the image of their Creator and share, as God's servants, in His kingly rule. As God's representatives in the creaturely realm, they are stewards of God's creatures. They are not to exploit, waste or despoil them, but to care for them and to use them in the service of God and humankind."

We are made in God's likeness; therefore, we represent Him.

We are God's ambassadors and are made to rule over livestock, birds, fish, and creatures that move along the ground. We have been given everything that lives and moves for food, but we are not to abuse them. Here is where we have gone wrong with our food system. The nutritional value between animals raised in a farmer's care, in his own field, and the animals raised in factory-type settings is very different. Fresh and home-prepared meats, vegetables, and cheeses nourish our bodies. Meat from confined, sickly animals does not. As we abuse animals by raising them in factory-like conditions, they diminish in their ability to nourish us. As we wander away from our role as caretakers, we also walk away from His blessing. Lest we forget, we are dependent on God's design. God is truly smarter than us.

> *Psalm 8:4-9 "What is man that you are mindful of him, the son of man that you care for him? You made him a little lower than the heavenly beings and crowned him with glory and honor. You made him rule over the works of your hands; you put everything under his feet: all flocks and herds, and beasts of the field, the birds of the air, and the fish of the sea, all that swim the paths of the seas. O Lord, our Lord, how majestic is your name in all the earth!"*

THE SONG OF MOSES

If we have been given everything for food, what can we use as a guideline for eating healthy? In Deuteronomy 32 there is a fascinating passage about the Lord God nourishing the people of Israel. It is interesting because the Lord spells out the kinds of food that He used to nourish them. This verse takes place toward the end of Deuteronomy, the last of the five books written by Moses, when he is standing before the promised land and is about to hand over the nation of Israel to Joshua. Moses stands before the nation of Israel and makes this speech beginning in verse 1:

> "Listen, O heavens, and I will speak; hear, O earth, the words of my mouth. Let my teaching fall like rain and my words descend like dew, like showers on new grass, like abundant rain on tender plants. I will proclaim the name of the Lord. Oh, praise the greatness of our God! He is the Rock, his works are perfect, and all his ways are just. A faithful God who does no wrong, upright and just is he..."

He charges the people with being unfaithful to their Creator and asks them to remember what God has done for them in the past. He goes on in verse 9:

> "For the Lord's portion is his people, Jacob his allotted inheritance. In a desert land he found him [the nation of Israel] in a barren and howling waste. He shielded him and cared for him; he guarded him as the apple of his eye, like an eagle that stirs up its nest and hovers over its young, that spreads its wings to catch them and carries them on its pinions."

Moses goes on to describe how the Lord nourished the nation of Israel in verse 12:

> "The Lord alone led him; no foreign god was with him. He made him ride on the heights of the land and fed him with the fruit of the fields. He nourished him with honey from the rock, and oil from the flinty crag, with curds and milk

> from herd and flock and with fattened lambs and
> goats, with choice rams of Bashan and the finest
> kernels of wheat. You drank the foaming blood
> of the grape. Jeshurun grew fat and kicked; filled
> with food, he became heavy and sleek."

Let's look at this in a little more detail, because when I first read this, I had no idea what "oil from the flinty crag" meant. The first and most important part is verse 12. God alone took care of Israel and there was no other god before them. They were completely dependent on the Lord, and he took care of their every need. In verse 13, where God "...fed him with the fruit of the fields. He nourished them with honey from the rock and oil from the flinty crag", my Bible's footnotes are very helpful here. It says that in Canaan, bees often built their hives in rocky crevices, and that olive trees often grew on rocky hillsides, such as the Mount of Olives just east of Jerusalem (If you do not have a study Bible, I highly recommend it! The footnotes are wonderful for putting Scripture into context and explaining details).

Basically, the Lord nourished them with the fruit (or "increase" -KJV) from the field, honey, olive oil, milk, curdled milk, fattened lambs and goats, choice sheep, wheat, and wine. The fruit or increase of the field could be anything from fruits, nuts, vegetables, grain, or field crops to animals that graze in fields (their young could be considered the "increase of the field"). Honey and olive oil are pretty specific, but "curdled milk" could be any type of fermented or soured milk such as butter, buttermilk, cheese, kefir, clabber, soft cheeses, yogurt, and whey. All are nutritious. If homemade from fresh milk and unpasteurized, they also provide many beneficial enzymes and bacteria that promote a healthy gut and digestive tract.

Two types of meat are listed here with details that they were fattened lambs and choice rams. The King James Bible says, "fat of lambs." I don't think it matters what type of animal we eat today, as God declared to Noah that He gave us all the earth for food (Genesis 9:3). In defense of red meat and healthy animal fats, I want to point out that God specifically listed fattened animals as one of the foods He gave to nourish the nation of Israel. I would assume that they used every part of the animal, such as the meat, fat, organs, marrow, and bones to make bone broths.

Wheat is listed, as well as the "foaming" blood of the grape, which I find very interesting. If you take a closer look at the process of wine making, the natural fermentation of the juice makes bubbles. This is bacteria breaking down the sugar in the juice and converting it to alcohol. The process of making vinegar is similar to winemaking. There is one more step required to convert the alcohol into vinegar. For example, balsamic vinegar is made from grapes. There are many drinks that have a special combination of yeasts and bacteria that convert sugars into alcohol, then into vinegar, releasing carbon dioxide and naturally making the drink fizzy like a soda. Sometimes these bacteria grow side-by-side in the same drink, with the end product being a vinegary-type drink, such as kombucha, which is an acidic, tart, but fizzy and flavorful drink. If unpasteurized, these drinks can supply a diverse abundance of beneficial yeasts and bacteria. They are living foods as well. "Fizzy" lemonade or homemade sodas can be made from lactic acid fermentation at home in your own kitchen. Lacto-fermentation can be used to make homemade root beer, sodas, water kefir, and things like lacto-fermented pickles.

Moses ends the song with a plea for the nation to remember his words and teach them to future generations. Deuteronomy 32:46 "...he said to them, 'Take to heart all the words I have solemnly declared to you this day, so that you may command your children to obey carefully all the words of this law. They are not idle words for you – they are your life. By them you will live long in the land you are crossing the Jordan to possess." We can remember how God fed and nourished the nation of Israel and teach these things to our children. It is God alone that provides for us.

Section Two
GOD'S DESIGN

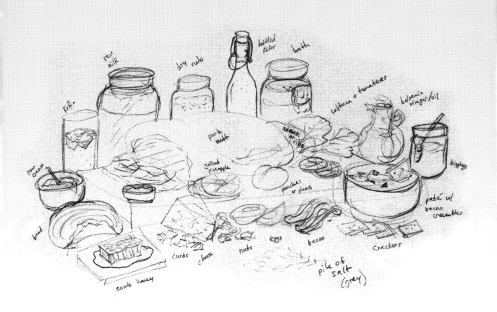

CAREFUL OBSERVATION PROVES GOD'S DESIGN

If God has given us everything for food, why are so many people sick? Because we are ignorant about God's design of our food. We are not asking the right questions and we're not asking enough questions. Let me introduce to you two words, "genetics" and "epigenetics." Genetics are God's design, or blueprint, for our bodies. It is the DNA or blueprint for how our bodies build themselves. Epigenetics are impacted by the environment the person is living in, what they eat, etc. I believe the chronic health problems we face today are due to epigenetics. The environment plays a big role in epigenetics. You can have a great blueprint to build a house but have a lousy environment. Epigenetics works like this: You give a contractor a blueprint to build a house, but instead of giving him concrete, lumber, and nails to work with you give him silly putty, popsicle sticks, and staples. The result will be a mess. Nutrition and taking care of our bodies is no different. Epigenetics is what your body has available to build itself with – it's impacted by your diet and what you eat. What happens when a civilization tosses their beef, butter, and whole grains and replaces them with fast food, margarine, and soft drinks? God's design becomes a mess. Thankfully, we have carefully documented observations about what happens to such civilizations that began to walk away from fresh food and replace them with modern foods.

EARLY WARNING SIGNS

In the early 1900s the world was changing rapidly. Trains and steam-powered boats were bringing goods for trade to cities and remote

What happens when a civilization tosses their beef, butter, and whole grains and replaces them with fast food, margarine, and soft drinks? God's design becomes a mess.

villages. There were only a handful of "modern" processed foods available. There was white (refined) flour, white (refined) sugar, canned condensed milk, and canned vegetables. Groups of people living in remote areas would come down to trading posts and trade for these grocery items.

A dentist by the name of Dr. Weston A. Price began to notice a difference in the health of people that began trading and consuming these early processed foods. He began to wonder why people living in areas too remote for trade had straight teeth, broad dental palates, resistance to disease, and ease of child birth while those living near trading posts who had access to modern foods began to decline rapidly in their health. Traveling to these remote regions to study the effects of adopting modern foods became his life's work. In 1939 he published his findings in a book, *Nutrition and Physical Degeneration*. His research came at a crucial time in history when modern medicine had not yet developed the ability to mask the complications of processed foods, as is common today with orthodontics and c-sections. Dr. Price and his wife traveled to the furthest and most remote villages to study those people who did not have access to modern foods and also studied what happened when family members moved closer to trading posts and port cities where modern foods could be found.

His observations are fascinating and heartbreaking. Of the children in the Loetschental Valley, Switzerland, he writes, "The sturdiness of the child life permits children to play and frolic bareheaded and barefooted even in water running down from the glacier in the late evening's chilly breezes, in weather that made us wear our overcoats and gloves and button our collars. Of all the children in the valley still using the primitive diet of whole rye bread and dairy products the average number of cavities per person was 0.3 per cent. On average it was necessary to examine three persons to find one defective deciduous or permanent tooth."[16] Their nutrition consisted of rye, used almost exclusively as a freshly ground cereal, dairy products from goats, and meat about once a week with a few green foods that were available during the summer.

As Dr. Price and his wife journeyed to villages with modern foods, the effects of processed foods became alarmingly visible.

> Nearby the Loetschental Valley, a village had a roadway built several years before Dr. Price and his wife visited the area. In this village canned and refined foods had been available for some time, and 20.2 percent of the children's teeth had been attacked by cavities. Other villages had the same symptoms. Practically every child had tooth decay. "Immediately one sees something is different here than in the primitive localities: the children have not the splendidly developed features, and the people give no evidence of the great physical reserve that is present in the smaller communities." Here, they shipped in modern white flour and had a bakery for sweetened baked goods, fruit jams, and jellies. "Usually it is not long after tunnels and roads are built that automobiles and wagons enter with modern foods, which begin their destructive work."

In his study of tribes of Northern Canada and the Yukon Territory, Dr. Price found these tribes were nomadic and wandering, following the herds of moose and caribou for food. The people were strong, free from disease, and had straight teeth. They had wide dental arches and cavities at only 0.16 percent. "The rigorous winters reach seventy degrees below zero. This precludes the possibility of maintaining dairy animals or growing seed cereals or fruits."[2] Their diet was almost entirely limited to wild hunted animals. Studying the nearby villages with access to processed foods, he found the percentage of cavities went up to 40 percent, with a marked increase in arthritis and tuberculosis. He did not find one case of arthritis in the remote tribes without processed foods.

In Africa, thirteen remote tribes were studied in which every individual had beautiful straight teeth and "superb physical health." Numerous other tribes were studied as well who had excellent teeth and wide dental palates. They depended on freshwater fish from lakes and rivers and dried them in the sun. They also made great use of corn, beans, sweet potatoes, and bananas. In Australia, the Aborigines were found to have great health, wide dental palates, and straight teeth as well. They hunted for wild game, ducks, and fish. Again, as they adopted modern processed foods their health began to decline rapidly.

Of the North American tribes, the same was also found. Many remote tribes were found with outstanding health, but tribes with access to trading posts developed deficiencies. Dr. Price writes, "A typical mother was studied at her home. She had four children. Her teeth were ravaged by dental caries. Twenty of her teeth had active caries. Her little girl, age four, already had twelve very badly carious teeth. Another daughter aged eight had sixteen carious teeth, and her son aged ten had six. The husband was in bed from acute lung involvement, doubtless tuberculosis. The children were eating their noon day meal when we arrived, which consisted of a white bread and some stewed vegetables. Milk was available for only the baby in arms. In this Tuscarora group, 83 per cent of those examined had dental caries. Every one studied in this reservation was using white-flour products, none was using milk liberally... They were now buying their wheat in the form of white-flour and their vegetables largely put up in cans. In both reservations, they were using commercial vegetable fats, jams and marmalades, sweetened goods, syrups and confections very liberally. It is remarkable how the child life adopts modern civilization's confections."

Processing food affects more than just cavities and disease

resistance. Women of many tribes, including the North American tribes and Eskimos, were known for their ease of childbirth and their ability to rear strong, rugged babies. There is a correlation between having a wide dental palate and having wide pelvic bones. Women who ate nutrient dense foods had wide dental arches, straight and beautiful teeth, and the ability to birth children easily. Dr. Price writes of the Eskimo women that "The women are characterized by the abundance of breastfood which almost always develops normally and is maintained without difficulty for a year. The mothers were completely free of dental caries, and I was told that the children of the Eskimos have no difficulties with the cutting of their teeth." However, at a reservation in Ontario, Canada where modern foods were available, Dr. Price visited with Dr. Davis, the Director of the hospital of that district. Dr. Davis said that the function of the hospital had changed over the twenty-eight years he had worked there. After watching three generations of mothers, he had noticed that the grandmothers had birthed children with ease at home, but the young mothers were brought to the hospital, often after being in labor for days. The young mothers were not able to birth their children easily and often needed surgical help in order to make the birth possible.

Pages and pages of stories describing the malnutrition of people who switched to processed foods can be found in Dr. Price's observations. He found the results consistent in all the remote groups he studied: the Swiss, Scottish, Eskimos, Native American tribes of Alaska and remote regions in the United States, the Seminole tribes of the Florida Everglades, Pacific Island tribes, Australian Aborigines, African tribes, the New Zealand Maori, and many others. As the remote people groups began trading and buying modern foods, their health began to deteriorate.

Let's not miss the amazing idea here: You can eat any food God has created and properly nourish your body. What I find fascinating is the broad spectrum of diets studied by Dr. Price and his wife. One village ate mostly rye bread and fresh cheese with meat only once a week, another village ate almost entirely seafood. One tribe was discovered to eat principally moose and deer meat, fresh fish and dried fish with a few vegetables when they were available. Island tribes ate seafood, wild pigs, various fruits and vegetables. These remote groups were eating fresh food, unprocessed and unadulterated: fresh milk and cheese from healthy grazing animals, roasted meats with all the juices and fats from roasting, dried meats and fruits, fresh ground grains, and used natural preservation to store their foods.

The only thing Dr. Price did not find was a group that ate only fruits and vegetables. He wrote that it was "a matter of keen interest, and at the same time disappointment since one of the purposes of the expedition to the South Seas was to find, if possible, plants or fruits, which together, without the use of animal products, were capable of providing all the requirements of the body." He searched, but did not find, any group that could sustain themselves on plants alone. Animal foods are essential to health: meat, eggs, seafood, poultry, bone broths, organ meats, and dairy products. But their nourishing abilities are lost when they are manipulated by modern processing.

A STORY OF HOPE

Here's the best part – some of those people left behind their canned and refined foods and returned to their former diet of whole, fresh food. In those cases, their dental caries were not active anymore and showed healing. The majority of people who returned to their nutrient-dense fresh foods began to recover from their afflictions. One example I find particularly useful is this story of a school for boys and girls on a North American reservation. This school, the Mohawk Institute, kept a fine dairy herd and provided fresh vegetables, whole wheat bread, and limited the sugar and white flour consumption of its students. Dr. Price did not find a single case of active caries among those he examined and attributed their health to the Institute's fine nutrition program. The children at the Institute had previous caries, but they were beginning to heal while eating the nutrient dense foods the Institute provided.

There is another study that closely parallels Dr. Price's research. Dr. Pottenger conducted several experiments with cats, studying the effects of cooked and pasteurized foods versus fresh milk and meat. His studies revealed similar effects. His control group of cats were fed fresh milk and meat. The second group of cats were fed pasteurized milk and cooked meat. By the second generation the cats fed pasteurized milk had developed all kinds of symptoms, including changes in facial structure, poor bone development, allergies, and degenerative disease.[17] By the fourth generation, the cats gave birth to stillborn or sterile young kittens that were not able to reproduce. Dr. Pottenger then did something unexpected. He took the second generation of sickly cats and put them back on the healthy diet of the control group cats. Within four generations, the new cats were as healthy as the control group cats.

Dr. Price's research proves God's design for nutrition is all we need. We don't need

> Within four generations, the new cats were as healthy as the control group cats.

to count calories or avoid entire foods groups in order to be healthy. Dr. Pottenger's research shows us God's grace. God has truly given us everything we need for nutrition, and when we return to His design we begin to heal. It is encouraging to me that God designed a world where people can eat foods native to their area, whether it is seafood or grazing animals, and glean all the nourishment the human body requires. Salt, minerals, and naturally fermented foods are also a part of this recipe and we will discuss them in detail. I am encouraged to know that we can change our diet and go back to nutrient dense foods and heal our bodies. Our children and grandchildren will be better for it. Let me challenge you to think about your food differently. Instead of asking, "What food group does it fall into," or "How many grams of fat or carbs does it contain," ask questions about where the food came from. Ask, "How was the animal raised and what was it fed? Was the animal healthy? How was the meat or plant processed? Was it pasteurized? Does it contain lab-created additives?" If you can't easily recreate it in your own kitchen, it's time to eat something else.

GOD'S LIVING FOODS: A HIDDEN WORLD

There are so much good bacteria that live all around us. It is easy for us to take them for granted. The truth is we cannot function without them. For years we were taught that our stomach acid and enzymes digest our food and that our stool is leftover food our body didn't use. However, this is far from the truth. New DNA sequencing "microscopes" have enabled scientists at the Human Microbiome Project to see how much living microorganisms are actually in our gut. They were astonished with what they found:

> "For years, bacteria have had a bad name. They are the cause of infections, of diseases. They are something to be scrubbed away, things to be avoided. But now researchers have taken a detailed look at another set of bacteria that may play even bigger roles in health and disease: the 100 trillion good bacteria that live in or on the human body. No one really knew much about them. They are essential for human life, needed to digest food, to synthesize certain vitamins, to form a barricade against disease-causing bacteria. But what do they look like in healthy people, and how much do they vary from person

to person? In a new five-year federal endeavor, the Human Microbiome Project, which has been compared to the Human Genome Project, 200 scientists at 80 institutions sequenced the genetic material of bacteria taken from nearly 250 healthy people. They discovered more strains than they had ever imagined — as many as a thousand bacterial strains on each person. And each person's collection of microbes, the microbiome, was different from the next person's. To the scientists' surprise, they also found genetic signatures of disease-causing bacteria lurking in everyone's microbiome. But instead of making people ill, or even infectious, these disease-causing microbes simply live peacefully among their neighbors... In adults, the body carries two to five pounds of bacteria, even though these cells are minuscule — one-tenth to one-hundredth the size of a human cell. The gut, in particular, is stuffed with them."[18]

The gut is not packed with food, it is stuffed full of microbes.[19] Some of these microbes your body can make, but many of them come from what we eat. About half of your stool is microbial mass, not leftover food. These bacteria also help the immune system.[20,21]

Where does all of the good bacteria come from? God designed these beneficial bacteria to be in most of the foods we eat. This is one of the main reasons why factory-produced food no longer nourishes us. Food processing destroys all the beneficial bacteria. Let's take a closer look at the way God created our world and the foods where these good microbes are found.

> God designed these beneficial bacteria to be in most of the foods we eat.

Where can we find foods that are full of beneficial bacteria, or what I call "living foods"? Here is where we get to study God's design of our world up close. Many people have heard of the beneficial bacteria *acidophilus*. The Latin name of this bacteria is *lactobacillus acidophilus*. Acidophilus is only one of many species in the group *lactobacillus*. In other words, acidophilus has many cousins, perhaps thousands. Lactobacteria, including acidophilus and all of its cousins, can be found on every living tree, shrub, grass, or plant from about five feet tall and downward into the soil. Lactobacillus bacteria are also found in numerous quantities in the soil. They must be important if God put them everywhere our food is found!

These bacteria can do some amazing things. They digest the sugars naturally found in plants, fruits, and vegetables and in return release an acidic "vinegar" that keeps harmful pathogens away. Lacto-fermentation is a natural process in which vegetables can be packed in jars with a small amount of salt and stored without refrigeration for a very long time. Lactobacteria surrounds the vegetables releasing lactic acid slowly over time, making the liquid grow more acidic. Bad bacteria cannot survive in acidic environments. They are not able to survive to spoil the food. This process is a centuries-old method for making pickles, chutneys, and relishes before refrigeration became available. These foods actually *increase* in nutrient content while they are being stored because the beneficial bacteria are "pre-digesting" the vegetables, releasing the vitamins locked up in the plant's cells.[22] The result is "pickled" food and veggies that are easy to digest and loaded with nutrients and beneficial bacteria your body needs in order to digest the vegetables. By God's design, food and vegetables stored this way become healthier for us as they are stored. Isn't God amazing?

Plants are not the only place these amazing bacteria can be found. Milk from grazing animals is loaded with beneficial bacteria. Since grazing animals eat grass all day, they are picking up the microflora in the grass they eat. This passes through their digestive system into the milk they produce. This bacteria, along with enzymes such as lactase, are naturally found in large quantities in unpasteurized, fresh milk. Fresh milk is another one of God's little miracles. The bacteria naturally found in the milk gently digests the sugars in the milk releasing acid and slowly sours the milk into delicious foods such as sour cream, butter, buttermilk, cheese, and whey. These are easy to make, and I have made them all in my kitchen with little effort. When homemade from fresh milk, *all* of these foods also contain the beneficial bacteria that was originally in the milk. It is a delicious way to multiply the beneficial bacteria that your body needs in order to be properly nourished. These foods are also filled with healthy fats and should be consumed on a regular basis.

Lactobacteria also release carbon dioxide as they digest sugar and release lactic acid. This naturally carbonates the foods that are being fermented. You can make homemade sodas from fresh fruit. They have a refreshing tingle and fizz that many people find enjoyable. By fermenting small batches of fresh fruit or juice with water kefir, you can make homemade sodas, such as ginger or pineapple soda. Let your imagination explore the possibilities: blackberry soda, ginger soda, lemon spice (lemon with cinnamon or mint). These are great on a hot summer day and children love them.

> *Psalm 139:13-14 NIV "For you created my inmost being; you knit me together in my mother's womb. I praise you because I am fearfully and wonderfully made; your works are wonderful, I know that full well."*

If raw milk isn't for you

If you don't feel comfortable buying raw milk, you have many options available to get living foods into your diet. Try experimenting with some of these foods. There is an entire chapter on Living Foods in Section Three, Understanding Your Food, where we will discuss how to make each food in detail.

Lacto-fermented vegetables: A method of making pickles and chutneys with either salt or whey before vinegar became the primary commercial way to make pickles. These are naturally fermented and tart, and they contain many probiotic and beneficial bacteria. They can be made dairy-free.

Water kefir: A homemade "soda" that can be made from any juice or fresh fruit. The kefir grains are similar to milk kefir grains, but thrive on natural sugars. They convert sugar into a mild vinegary-tart drink. They can be sweetened afterwards by adding more juice. By using air lock lids, you can create the same amount of carbonation as store-bought sodas. Grape juice produces a homemade soda that tastes exactly like sparkling grape juice. Some tasty options are strawberry soda, apple cinnamon soda, grape soda, pineapple ginger, etc. They have a wide variety of beneficial bacteria and yeasts. I think these drinks are the most mild and easiest for families new to living foods. They are more mild than kombucha and they are also dairy-free.

Kombucha: Stronger than water kefir, most kombucha takes a little getting used to. Sweet-tart and fizzy, kombucha is carbonated and full of beneficial bacteria, especially lactobacillus coagulans, the primary ingredient in Digestive Advantage, a probiotic gummy. One benefit, however, is that kombucha can be purchased at most Publix and Target stores in the produce section. If they are too strong for you, they can also be mixed with juice to dilute the tart flavor. You can buy kombucha in many different flavors, but my personal favorite is GT's Strawberry Kombucha.

Milk kefir: Milk kefir grains are wonderful to work with and make a thin yogurt-like drink, but without all the fuss. Milk kefir also has a wide variety of beneficial bacteria and yeasts, more so than water kefir. If you don't want raw milk, start with pasteurized milk from grass-fed cows and add the kefir grains. After culturing, pour off the kefir, saving the grains to be used again. You can add fruit and flavors to your kefir to make all kinds of tasty options.

Yogurt: Yogurt is a great living food, but if buying commercially prepared yogurt, try to find a yogurt that is full-fat and contains at least several different strains of beneficial bacteria. These should be listed on the label. The temptation with yogurt is to buy the super-sweetened varieties with cookies and chocolate that are more like a dessert than yogurt. Just keep an eye on how much sugar you're eating.

LIVING FOODS AND THE AUTO-IMMUNE SYSTEM

To appreciate how important it is to eat living foods, you must understand how the immune system works. Here's where God's design really shines. Most bad bacteria cannot survive in acidic environments. Pathogens that enter the mouth are first met with an acidic environment. Stomach acid is the next line of defense, dropping in pH to a level of 4.0-5.0 near the gut wall.[23] If pathogens survive past the stomach into the gut, they are then met with the bulk of the immune system where a whole host of beneficial bacteria are ready and waiting to keep pathogens in check.

In other words, a large portion of the immune system is found in the gut, or small intestine. Remember, the gut is stuffed with microbes, or beneficial bacteria. Dr. Natasha Campbell-McBride, founder of The Cambridge Nutrition Clinic and author of *Gut and Psychology Syndrome*, says of the immune system, "On the whole it is hard to overestimate how important the state of our gut flora is in the appropriate functioning of our immune system. It has been estimated that around 80-85% of our immunity is located in the gut wall. The gut wall with its bacterial layer can be described as the right hand of the immune system. If the bacterial layer is damaged or, worse than that, abnormal, then the person's immune system is trying to function with its right hand tied behind its back."

"Gut dysbiosis," or abnormal gut flora, is the result of poor diet, taking medicine for chronic pain, doses of antibiotics, stress, and other factors. Maintaining a poor diet, such as eating too much sugar or starchy foods, can cause an overgrowth of fungi and pathogens in the gut lining. These fungi and pathogens can excrete toxins into the gut that pass through the gut wall into the bloodstream. They wreak havoc on the immune system. Some fungi have roots shaped like spirals that can puncture the gut wall, creating holes and "leaky gut" syndrome.[24,25] These fungi feed on sugar and starches. Eating a diet high in sugar and starches encourages these fungi and pathogens to multiply, disturbing the balance of beneficial bacteria in the gut. Taking antibiotics or long-term use of aspirin, ibuprofen, or contraceptive pills can also cause gut flora imbalance.[26] To make matters worse, imbalanced gut flora can be passed from mother to child during childbirth and breastfeeding. On the other hand, *healthy* gut flora can also be passed from mother to child during childbirth and breastfeeding. That's one more reason why eating living foods and following God's design for nutrition during pregnancy and post-partum is vital to your child's health.

> Some fungi have roots shaped like spirals that can puncture the gut wall, creating holes and "leaky gut" syndrome. These fungi feed on sugar and starches.

Gut dysbiosis causes many imbalances and weaknesses in the integrity of the gut wall. Dr. Campbell-McBride explains that without the beneficial bacterial lining along the digestive tract viruses, fungi, and toxins get through the wall and into the bloodstream. The lack of beneficial bacteria allows opportunistic microflora to take over, disrupting the delicate balance of the gut. Many of these pathogens release toxins into the gut and in turn, damage the gut wall. A damaged, imbalanced gut wall can only partially digest food allowing partially digested foods to pass through the gut wall and into the blood stream. These partially digested foods are recognized as foreign objects and are then attacked by the immune system. This is how food allergies develop. A leaky gut wall lining does not absorb nutrients as well, further compounding the problem by allowing the body to become malnourished. This damaged system is not able to properly digest foods and nourish the body or keep pathogens in check.

The lack of beneficial bacteria in the gut causes a suppressed immune system and leaky gut wall, triggering overactive immune reactions. It creates a landscape of chronic viral infections, allergies, asthma, eczema, and many other chronic symptoms. When we do not eat the foods God designed to properly nourish our bodies, we end up with a damaged and leaky gut wall and a badly compromised immune system.

The good news is that a damaged gut wall can be healed by changing the foods your family eats. Getting sugary, starchy foods and cheap, junk food out of your diet may be challenging but replacing them with fresh, whole foods and delicious fats is fun and tasty! You can also reduce the damage from medicine and antibiotics by eating and drinking living foods full of beneficial bacteria.

> *Psalm 100:1-3 "Shout to the Lord, all the earth. Worship the Lord with gladness; come before him with joyful songs. Know that the Lord is God. It is he who made us, and we are his; we are his people, the sheep of his pasture."*

GUT AND COLON HEALTH

When I am not milking cows at home on our small farm, I am tending fruit trees and a small vegetable garden near the driveway. I've always had an interest in gardening and cooking. After all, the two hobbies go together very well. If you have a love for cooking delicious food, odds are, you also have a deep appreciation for fresh, great tasting fruit and vegetables. What better way to cook delicious food than to have a small garden patch just outside your kitchen door? It also turned out to be a great way to get my children to eat veggies because they loved the idea of growing "snacks" they could eat right in the yard.

As I began to learn about all the microflora in our digestive system, I began to notice some peculiar similarities between our guts and the soil. Many of the bacteria names were the same.

29

The beneficial bacteria I was working with in the kitchen to pickle vegetables was the same bacteria I was reading about in my gardening books. The same bacteria I needed to ferment milk was the same I needed to get my compost pile healthy. Much of the bacteria and soil life is the same as what is in our gut. It makes sense. Our food comes from the soil. Carrots are pulled up right out of the ground. Beasts of the field eat grass and munch soil-grown plants all day. Their milk is loaded with soil-borne microflora.

It began to bother me that so much of our food is sterilized and pasteurized. I was working so hard at home to preserve, multiply, and ferment foods that had beneficial life in them. These beneficial microflora help keep the body's internal plumbing working properly. I began to realize that the colon operates much like a compost pile. You see, for a compost pile to "compost" or break down organic material correctly, several ingredients are necessary: green material (fresh cut grass, leaves, or kitchen scraps), brown material (dry leaves, sticks, or hay), water, and microflora. Without water, a compost pile just sits there. The soil bacteria dies and everything turns brown and dry. Without a good mix of brown and green material, the microflora in the compost pile gets off balance. Too much brown, dry material and there is not enough "food" to support them. Too much green material and the beneficial flora gets out of balance, inviting fungus growth. Then the compost pile begins to smell foul.

Our guts are no different. They need green material (fresh food), brown material (fiber), water, and microflora. Without beneficial flora our guts cannot do the hard job of digesting the food in our intestines. The absence of microflora leads to constipation. This is easily remedied by adding fresh raw milk, lacto-fermented foods, or drinks such as kombucha or water kefir to the diet.

Without adequate water and fiber, the flora cannot multiply and have the environment they need to thrive. This also leads to constipation. Drinking enough water is so important. If your family cannot stand drinking plain water, try the fizzy homemade sodas in the recipe section, such as water kefir. They are full of water and beneficial bacteria. Also be aware that caffeine and sugary drinks are dehydrating. Drinking coffee, caffeinated tea, and sodas do not help but hurt a thirsty body. If you are going to drink these, follow with a large glass of water.

Fiber is found in many foods that God created. Most fresh fruit and vegetables contain fiber. Grains, beans and nuts are terrific sources of fiber! Want to know why beans sometimes cause gas? They contain so much fiber they cause a burst of flora production in our bowels. Any other time you add bacteria or yeast to something and expect it to grow (bread rising, lacto-fermented pickles, milk souring, grape juice fermenting), there are always air bubbles that are released as the beneficial bacteria do their work. They exhale just like any other life form. The gas that is experienced from beans is more than likely the bowels coming to life. It can be painful if there is too much gas, and for this reason, I always soak beans overnight until they swell and split their shells. They will double in size. Beans are seeds, after all. They are in a dormant state. Soaking overnight brings the seed back into its "awake" or plant-like stage, and makes it much easier to digest. You cannot do this with canned or cooked beans.

Too much processed food without microflora, which I would call junk food, leads to bacteria imbalance and foul smell; in other words, upset stomach and diarrhea. There are many things that can cause a flora imbalance in our gut, some of which are fast food, junk food, stomach flu, stress, and antibiotics. Thankfully, this is corrected by adding back into the diet beneficial flora as found in fresh unpasteurized milk, lacto-fermented foods, and living drinks such as kombucha or kefir. These living foods are wonderful for repopulating a digestive system that is struggling or under attack, such as by antibiotics or recovering from a stomach flu.

Psalm 62:5 "Find rest, O my soul, in God alone; my hope comes from him."

Easing into Living Foods

It's important to understand that when you first begin eating or drinking living foods, you must ease into them slowly. Living foods create gas when they first establish themselves in the gut. You will want to start with small amounts, such as 4-6 ounces of raw milk, kefir, or water kefir a day for the first several days until the beneficial microflora get established in the gut. Once established, they don't cause any noticeable gas.

A note about fiber: Eating a whole bunch of fiber, say a whole bowl of beans, and a tall glass of a living foods drink is also a bad idea in the beginning. Microflora need fiber to survive, but lots of fiber can encourage them to multiply rapidly, hence lots of gas. If beans and fiber (or high fiber energy bars) are already part of your regular routine, then just add living foods slowly into the diet a little bit at a time. As long as you do not feel any discomfort or gas pains after a day or so, then it is fine to add a bit more the following day.

OBESITY: A SYMPTOM OF MALNUTRITION

A person or child can starve from lack of food. Most everyone has seen photos of starving children in countries that are in dire need of food. These children are so thin it is painful to look at the photos. These conditions are caused by drought, war, natural disaster, lack of clean water, or economic difficulties. This is starvation by sheer lack of any type of food. Did you know that there is another way to starve? Let me ask you this: is it possible to be surrounded by food and still starve? To death, no, but what if it is possible to be surrounded by cheap food and starve your body of essential nutrition? What would that look like?

It would look like obesity. Remember when I said our nation is knee-deep in cheap food? This processed food is devoid of essential nutrients and enzymes that our bodies need in order to thrive. The result is a type of nutrition "famine" that brings on malnutrition. This malnutrition shows itself as obesity and chronic health problems. I want to make sure I explain this clearly – obesity is not caused by eating too much food. Yes, the Bible talks about gluttony, but that's not what we're talking about here. Obesity plagues Western civilization, and Western civilization is plagued by processed foods. Obesity is not caused by eating too much fat. It is caused by eating nutrient poor foods. Empty foods. Dead foods. It's not just vitamins that are missing. Enzymes and probiotic microflora in living foods are missing from processed foods. The heating and processing destroys them. Our bodies are not able to glean the nourishment they need to thrive from a TV dinner. If you are obese, will you allow me to free you from the guilt of eating too much food? There's a reason why those living in poverty in western civilization are typically obese. It's not because they eat too much food. The wealthy in Western civilization are typically thin. They can afford to buy steak and fresh leafy vegetables. It's not because they don't eat enough. Processed and subsidized foods are cheaper and more affordable in the United States. They are refined carbs, starches and snacks... exactly what leads to obesity. The solution is to find quality, nutrient-dense foods. There are many that are affordable; some you can even get for free.

My husband and I were most unhealthy when we were both working fulltime and eating out at restaurants frequently. We had little time to cook and bought many convenience foods. We had acid reflux, weight management issues, digestive problems, and very high cholesterol. At 25, my cholesterol was 199. We didn't feel healthy. All of that changed when we started eating and cooking at home. However, the changes we made were different compared to what is recommended today. According to our nation's food guidelines, we began eating very "unhealthy" foods. I saved the fat from our bacon and used that to deep fry our potatoes. We ate eggs every morning and I put heavy cream in my coffee. We drastically reduced the amount of sugar we were eating and stopped buying sodas. We began buying beef from a lady who raised beef locally. She gave us the liver, bones, and fat from the beef for free. I cooked the precious fat and saved the melted beef fat into jars. We used this beef fat, called tallow, to make gravies and roasts that would make anyone drool. I roasted the beef bones into delicious, rich broth. I cooked all our vegetables in butter or served fresh sliced veggies with creamy homemade dips. We bought a grain mill and began grinding our own fresh wheat for bread. We began making water kefir at home. You know what happened? Our cholesterol balanced, my husband stopped taking Prilosec, and we are healthier now than we have ever been. We have lost weight and I have gone down a dress size, but we are not weak from losing weight. We are strong and our immune systems are very healthy. I can't honestly tell you if we've caught many colds this year because they are difficult to tell apart from allergies. Mostly, we just sniffle and are tired for a day or two, then we are back to normal. Almost everything on our plates resembles the food it comes from: either meat, grains, fruits, or vegetables. I began to notice that very little of the food we purchased came in boxes, and the food we make at home tastes *so* much better.

Let me explain obesity by malnutrition in a little more detail. Processing food destroys the very nature of it. Our food is delicate. Years ago, I grew an interest in making homemade cheese. I bought milk at the store and ordered the necessary enzymes and rennet to curdle the milk and turn it into cheese. What I discovered is that you cannot use store-bought milk to make cheese. It has been heated to very high temperatures that denature the proteins in the milk. What you end up with is a pile of white mushy mess. In order to make homemade cheese you have to find milk that has not been pasteurized, or that has been heated only very little. Ultra-heat-treated milk, or UHT, has been pasteurized to such temperatures that the milk proteins are destroyed. This is what I call "dead milk." It is not a living food anymore.

Store-bought cereals that have been cooked, high-heat processed, and puffed out into little shapes do not nourish the body regardless of how many vitamins are added back into the final product. The life of the grain is gone. Whole grains fresh-milled are a far better option. They also contain no additives or conditioners.

By God's design, vitamins are naturally found in foods with the proper enzymes needed to digest those vitamins. For example, water-soluble vitamin C is naturally found in oranges with the natural enzymes needed in the orange. They are paired together. These enzymes are very fragile. Heat and processing destroys them. The enzymes in our food, especially raw foods or homemade foods, aid in digestion of our food. Foods high in enzymes reduce the body's need to create these enzymes, lightening the work load on the pancreas. Enzymes are deactivated at a wet-heat temperature of 118 degrees Fahrenheit. By God's design, the human body can safely touch foods and liquids at 117 degrees or lower.[27] God has given us a built-in mechanism for determining whether or not we are overcooking our foods. Isn't that wonderful? It just so happens that most homemade cheeses are also heated at 110 degrees or less. This allows homemade, fresh-milled foods to be much higher in vitamin and enzyme content. Homemade foods are nutrient dense, easier to digest, and far better in flavor.

Pasteurized, concentrated orange juice with added vitamin C is not the same quality as eating a fresh orange off the tree.

Yet, this is how our food is marketed and sold. Juice boxes for children are labeled with such things as "Equivalent to two servings of fruit" No, it's not! Don't be fooled. One substance that does survive the processing of juice is sugar. Have you ever tried to juice an apple? It would take several apples to make one cup of juice. This does not mean that a cup of juice is equal to several fresh, sliced apples off the tree. It means that cup of juice is equal to the sugar content of several apples. Our families do not need that much sugar. We would be far better off planting fresh fruit trees in parks and around our homes. Can't grow citrus where you live? That's okay, plant blueberries. Plant plums or figs. Tropical areas can grow guava and mangoes. Ever notice that all fruit seems to be high in the same vitamins? God did not put all the vitamins needed for survival in one type of fruit. Don't believe advertising that suggests one superfood is the only source of a needed vitamin.

Look around and see what foods are native to your area and visit your local farmer's market. Don't be afraid of healthy animal fats, especially if they are from local, small farms. Farmer's markets are a gold mine for local, fresh food. Yes, they may cost more, but remember you are paying people for the real cost of producing food. This creates jobs where farmers can be paid fairly for their hard work. Think about how much money you will save on medicine and antacids!

IMMUNE SYSTEM CRISIS

We've seen in the last several decades an explosion of "unexplainable" symptoms in the health of children and adults. We are witnessing an alarming increase of children with allergies to what used to be everyday foods: milk, nuts, wheat, fruit, etc. What's going on? Children are increasingly diagnosed with ADHD and autism. Adult cases increase of IBS, Crone's disease, Lyme disease... even to people who don't camp or who are exposed to ticks.

These all have something in common, what I call immune system shutdown or "crisis." When the immune system begins to suffer, it begins to show symptoms. Just like a car that needs a mechanic begins to clunk and make noise, our immune systems begin to show signs of damage. The symptoms, though, are different in each person because of the way the immune system operates. Let me explain. Remember the discovery that the Human Microbiome Project discovered – that there are pathogens and diseases lurking in everyone's gut, but that our beneficial microflora in the gut hold these pathogens in check? What happens when these beneficial microflora begin to fail? Any number of pathogens or opportunistic microflora can begin to multiply and dominate over our own beneficial flora, and gut dysbiosis, or imbalance, sets in.

For example, ten different people can take multiple rounds of antibiotics for an infection, say... a chronic urinary tract infection. Antibiotics reduce the amount of beneficial microflora in the gut as they also reduce the amount of the infection in the urinary tract. Those ten people's immune systems are compromised by the antibiotics, but will each show different symptoms. One may develop chronic constipation due to lack of beneficial microflora in the gut, another may develop diarrhea, another may develop IBS, and another may catch colds and stomach bugs easier for the next six months until their immune systems restore their beneficial microflora. Still, another person may develop Lyme disease because the pathogen was already in the gut, but is now no longer being held in check by beneficial microflora. Also, another person develops "leaky gut" as the microflora get out of balance and bacteria develop in the gut with roots that pierce the stomach and gut wall, causing small lesions in the gut lining. This leads to partially undigested food passing through the gut wall into the bloodstream, causing what we know today as food allergies.

There is *very* good news! We are "fearfully and wonderfully made." Our immune systems can repair themselves and the damage

> God's living foods restore the balance of beneficial microflora.

can be healed. It can be healed! And we can help our immune systems by eating foods the way God created them. God's living foods restore the balance of beneficial microflora. We can choose to eat a portion of living foods every day, giving help to our bodies and healing the gut. Our bodies know what to do. And the best part is, if your doctor says you need antibiotics, you can take them along with living foods and lessen the damage to your gut and immune system. God has given us grace, but we must choose to follow His design.

Let me show you in a little more detail what immune system crisis looks like. When we hear things like "rare infection, Lyme disease, IBS, immune disorders," that should send a red flag to us to start augmenting and fortifying the immune system. The medical establishment is trained to track down and eliminate specific diseases or pathogens. Individually, this works, but not when the problem is systematic. When the immune system begins to fail, eliminating one pathogen will only work for a while before another pathogen surfaces because it is also not being held in check by beneficial microflora. It's impossible to fight each one independently. Multiple rounds of antibiotics only weaken the immune system further by destroying more of the beneficial microflora. The best approach is to begin augmenting and nourishing the immune system and healing the gut lining so that beneficial microflora can resume their work of holding pathogens in check.

How do we know if the immune system is functioning properly? It is good to have clear, traceable numbers and distinct diagnosis in the medical field. How can we measure the immune system? If the clearest descriptor of a healthy immune system is the absence of disease, how do we measure that? That's difficult to track. In a healthy system, the pathogens are already in the gut, they're just kept in check. Healthy gut microflora will show pathogens in the microbiome, but the patient will not show any signs of symptoms. As the immune system begins to fail, due to poor diet, gut dysbiosis, medications, etc., we will see symptoms of immune system failure begin to emerge.

Symptoms of a Sinking Immune System

		Possible Causes
Healthy — healthy, rarely catches colds, daily bowel movement	healthy gut flora	daily living foods / whole foods diet
Suffering — occasional constipation		processed foods
nutrient deficeintcies develop	gut dysbiosis	lack of living food
multiple allergies		junk food
regular constipation, constant nasal drip		mediciations
food allergies, leaky gut		the pill
Crisis — irritable bowel syndrome, Lyme disease	gut failure	multiple rounds of antibiotics
frequent bowel cramping and diarreaha after eating		multiple medications
rare bacterial infections		painkillers

This chart shows the meltdown process of the human immune system. At the top is the healthy person with a fully functioning microbiome full of beneficial microflora. They are healthy, rarely catch colds, have no allergies, and no constipation or diarrhea. As poor diet sets in, gut health declines from junk food, fast food, and lack of living foods to replenish the immune system.

Over time, nutrient deficiencies develop and beneficial microflora declines. The immune system is suffering at this point, but still able to keep the person looking healthy at first glance. Subtle symptoms begin to emerge such as seasonal allergies and chronic constipation. Further down the chart, well into the suffering category, are those who have had to take painkillers or other medications that damage the gut lining. For some people, leaky gut or food allergies begin to develop.

At the bottom of the chart is where immune system failure or "crisis" begins to happen. Multiple rounds of antibiotics can weaken the immune system to the point that some begin to develop IBS, Crone's, or Lyme disease and the gut lining begins to fail. Some people actually develop lesions in the gut lining. Frequent gut cramping, chronic diarrhea, and rare bacterial infections emerge. These people need immediate help in healing the gut and immune system.

Climbing Out of the Well: Healing the Gut and Immune System

Healthy		simple starches roast potatoes	healthy gut flora	whole foods living foods
Suffering		turbinado or raw sugar home-milled breads	gut dysbiosis	limited starches some sweeteners
Crisis		living foods drinks for gut health bone broth, cooked down vegetables in broth honey, raw milk, milk or water kefir, sea salt farm fresh eggs, butter, roasted meat	gut failure	living foods nutrient dense foods very little sweeteners

For those who are in immune system crisis, the GAPS diet developed by Dr. Natasha Campbell McBride is outstanding in walking a patient through the steps of healing a failing gut. She outlines a plan, based on nutrient-dense and easy-to-digest foods, that stops the irritation to the gut and begins to restore proper function of the immune system. These steps should be followed under a doctor's guidance and with the help of family members to help prep and create meals that soothe and nourish the gut lining. Bone broths rich in gelatin, carefully cooked down meat and vegetables, and living foods help to heal the gut.

For those who fall under the category of suffering immune systems, increasing the amount of living foods in the diet is an excellent way to begin nourishing the immune system. Staying away from processed foods and focusing on whole, fresh foods is tasty, delicious, and will reap many rewards for those who take the time to prepare them.

For those who are blessed to live in the healthy category, eating a small amount of living foods once a day, or definitely when you feel a cold coming on will help maintain the balance of beneficial microflora in your system.

LOSING WEIGHT AND BALANCING BLOOD SUGAR

The false notion that eating fat causes obesity – and the equally false notion of burning calories to lose weight – is so ingrained in American culture that anyone who thinks otherwise must be completely crazy. The truth is actually good news and far more tasty. True, exercise will help strengthen muscles and help a person feel better. Exercise is good for the body. It builds muscle, body tone, and strengthens the body core. False, eating less will not help a person lose weight - not permanently. Eating less while eating nutrient poor foods can be a disaster for the body. Eating a nutrient poor diet combined with extreme exercising can be downright dangerous. It starves the body while pushing it to burn large amounts of energy, but without replacing the needed fuel. Animal fats are long-burning fuels that do not raise blood sugar levels.

The body depends on two primary sources of fuel for energy: carbs and fats. Carbohydrates are a necessary fuel that creates a short burst of energy. The body burns through them very quickly. They are especially helpful in restoring energy after a fever or sickness. Fats are slow burning and help balance blood sugar levels. They pair especially well with natural sugars. Historically, many desserts have been a rich and simple pairing of fats, cream, and natural sugars. Fats are necessary to balance the insulin rush from the sugar in the dessert. Sugar eaten on a low-fat diet causes an insulin rush with no long-burning fats to help stabilize blood sugar levels. The result is a mighty crash that leaves the person feeling tired, shaky, and craving more fuel... any kind of fuel, especially a quick-burning sugar rush to bring blood sugar levels back up to where they are supposed to be. But snacking on sugars and starches does not last long, so the body is caught in a roller coaster ride trying to balance blood sugar levels and energy crashes and spikes. Eating a low-fat and low-carb diet leaves the body with no fuel at all. To lose weight, it is far better to skip the sugar all together and eat healthy animal fats, proteins, and quality carbs like fresh fruits and vegetables. A breakfast of scrambled eggs in butter with fresh sliced apples will hold energy levels, burning slowly through until lunch time. No crashes, no cravings. Skip the waffles and skip the sugar. Eat bacon or sausage with yogurt.

To make matters worse, low-fat foods like salad dressing typically add more sugar to make up for the lost flavor from reducing fat. A breakfast of low-fat cereal with skim milk (which is almost all sugar) will leave a person starving by mid-morning. If they worked out that morning, the body is already at an energy deficit and craving a quality source of energy. A mid-morning piece of candy only spikes blood sugar levels and leaves it to crash about thirty minutes later, so by 11:30 the person is tired, shaky and wondering why he or she cannot focus on their work. Lunch for many dieting people is a "hearty" salad with low-fat dressing. The lettuce, veggies, some cheese (which helps), and sugary salad dressing do not help balance blood sugar or provide the quality fuel they need. Most people continue on this roller coaster ride of snacking and energy crashes throughout the day. The energy crash caused by eating sugar with no fats is not helped by drinking coffee. This helps explain why many people come home exhausted at the end of the day, even if they work at a desk job.

To lose weight, you cannot ride the blood sugar roller coaster. You need to eat the highest quality fuels for your body, along with a healthy portion of living foods. Breakfast has to include a hearty portion of protein and animal fats. Commercial oatmeal and cereal are highly refined grains, most of which offer little nutritional value. They are empty carbs. It's fine to eat some oatmeal with buttered eggs and bacon, but the healthy fats must be there to offset the sugar crash that will be caused by the oatmeal or cereal.

If blood sugar levels drop, eat a high-protein and fat snack. Peanuts (not sugar coated or candied) and peanut butter make a great snack fuel. Beef jerky is another good snack, although it is usually too lean to provide much fuel. Salami or sausage, which contain a higher percentage of fat, is a better choice. So are hard boiled eggs (with the yolk), tuna salad with an oily sauce (like coconut oil with a little mustard and lemon juice). Full fat yogurt is another good choice. Skip the yogurt with cookie crumbles on top and go for the whole milk vanilla yogurt. It contains far less sugar and more fats to last through the day.

Keep in mind which weather season you are currently in. Summer snacks and meals can be lighter, with more fruit and watery foods such as watermelon. When temperatures rise in midsummer heat, the body shifts its energy to sweating and cooling the body. Lighter foods such as grilled chicken and veggies or seafood are perfect for hot summer days. Winter meals need to be higher in fat. The body needs those long burning fuels to keep up body temperature. Winter meals have traditionally been heavier for that reason. Meals such as roasted meats with gravy, thick hearty (and oily) soups, chili and smoked sausages are perfect for days when it's snowing outside.

Family meals, such as lunch and dinner, are perfect for working in the much-needed fruit and veggies, along with protein and fats. Sour cream, olive and coconut oils are great for dips and sauces. When it comes to preparing lunch, sometimes the best thing to do is cook a really large dinner the night before and pack the leftovers for lunch. I'm not talking about cold pizza. Roast a whole chicken with veggies in the crock pot while you are at work. Have that for supper, then pack leftovers for tomorrow's lunch. Pulled bits of chicken from the frame, along with whatever gravy and juices collected in the bottom of the crock pot, makes a great lunch. You get meat, protein, fats, soft cooked veggies all together in an easy to fix lunch that can be eaten cold or hot. Add some fresh sliced fruit and a full fat creamy dip with veggies (especially if you have access to fresh, unpasteurized milk or cheese), and you have a full meal with living foods. We have a very large crock pot in our house that is the work horse of our kitchen. About every three days I'm putting something in the slow cooker, and I keep every scrap of juice and fat that cooks out of the meat.

Remember when I say "start cooking at home", I don't mean baking. There's a big difference between cooking and baking. Baking usually involves lots of sugar which is better to avoid when trying to lose weight. Think barbecue. Roasting, grilling, sautéing meats and vegetables and keep all the juice and fats that melt away from the meat. I store them in little jars in the fridge. They come in handy when there isn't enough time to slow cook and they add fat and flavor to a bag of flavorless frozen veggies.

Counting and Burning Calories

When it comes to losing weight, many people count calories and try to burn calories. There is the belief that as long as you burn more calories than you eat, you should be able to lose weight. If they are still unable to lose weight, they eat less and try to exercise more with the hope that they will burn more calories than they are consuming. I have a hard time believing that God would create a world where we need to count calories in order to stay trim and healthy. Part of the problem is the assumption that all calories are created equal. The other part of the problem is the belief that if you burn calories, you are burning *those same calories that make you fat* when you exercise.

Think about it for a moment: if scientists are still discovering what's inside our gut, then how can they possibly know exactly how our bodies are going to breakdown our food? How can they know that food X contains exactly X number of calories and exercising for X number of minutes will burn those same calories? That violates rule #1: Don't assume you know everything about God's creation. How can people possibly know that a glass of milk will be broken down and used the same way in adults versus children, in elderly versus teens, in women versus men, regardless to heredity, metabolism, and which season the person is living in? Is a carrot eaten by someone living in the tropics, sweating in the shade, processed the same way as a carrot eaten by a person who is living in an area buried in four feet of snow? Does a carrot grown in Florida sandy soil have the same nutritional value as one grown in Carolina clay soil? Because we don't know, *we can't base our entire diet around this wild assumption!*

USING EVERYTHING GOD HAS GIVEN US

To appreciate every part of an animal (and save money), it's important to understand how God designed the food he made for us. Every part of an animal is nutritious. The muscle meat, fat, bones, organs, joints, and ligaments all carry nutrition that can be assimilated by people and used to rebuild their bones and joints. The organs, such as liver, have been held in high regard in the past as being very nutritious. There are passages of scripture that talk about how animal fat was highly esteemed in the Old Testament. God himself said in Leviticus that the fat of sacrificed animals was not to be eaten, but set aside for the Lord, especially the fat around the liver and kidneys. "All the fat is the Lord's" (Leviticus 3)*. This animal fat was so highly prized that God claimed it as His own. The bones and joints of animals have traditionally been boiled for making bone broths.

To see how the average family wastes money, here's an example. A family of four can purchase chicken breast strips, soup, chicken salad, vegetable oil for frying, vitamins, glucosamine for better joints, and think that these items are not related. However, at our house, we purchase a whole chicken and use the leftovers to make all the items listed above. I roast the chicken in the oven on the first day, saving all the juices and liquid that cook out of the chicken. What's left is a chicken frame with little bits of meat that we pull from the frame and place in a freezer bag to be saved for chicken salad. Then, I place the chicken frame (and any fat or leftover skin) in the slow cooker, filling it with enough water to cover the bones. I add a teaspoon of apple cider vinegar or lemon juice, spices, sea salt, and let it cook on low for six hours or more. The bones, cartilage, and marrow become soft and begin to dissolve in the broth. This tasty bone broth is rich in vitamins and minerals. After simmering in the slow cooker, we have about a half-gallon of bone broth that I strain and store in the fridge.

Properly made bone broth (with joints and cartilage) gels in the fridge. The dissolved cartilage melts into the broth creating a rich and tasty broth, superior to any store-bought broth. The cartilage also becomes a natural gelatin, from which glucosamine is derived. When the broth gels, the fat also rises to the top and solidifies. I scoop this off and use it for mouth-watering gravies and sauces. You can cook any vegetable in roast chicken fat and it will taste amazing. I'm convinced that the reason people hate vegetables is because we have been taught to cook them without roasted animal fats. Vegetables need tasty fats. Chicken liver is also rich in minerals and vitamins. Our family is not used to the taste of liver, so we do not eat liver as a meal. We hide it in our food. I make Italian meatballs, chili, and tacos that have bits of liver in them, but the flavor is not noticeable in these strongly flavored foods. A family can justify paying a little more for a whole chicken when every bit of goodness is gleaned from it in this way.

*To prevent confusion, Leviticus 3 ends with the statement, "You must not eat any fat or blood." I have cross-referenced this verse many times and I believe that the Lord is speaking to the Israelites in this verse about the Fellowship Offering. It was the only offering in which the person may eat a portion. However, the fat of the Fellowship Offering was forbidden because "All the fat is the Lord's" v. 3:16. The fat was highly prized by God and was to be burned on the altar. There are many other places where the Bible speaks favorably of eating the fat of animals, such as Deuteronomy 32:14. The Bible even uses the term "fat" to mean abundance, health, and prosperity, ex: "the fat of the land."

Section Three
UNDERSTANDING FRESH FOOD

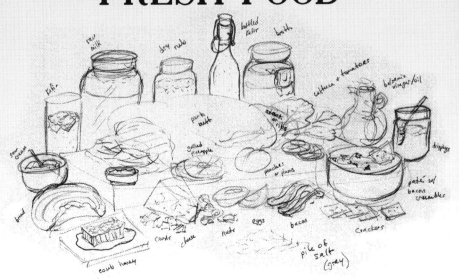

COOKING WITH FRESH FOOD

Welcome to the tasty section of this book! I love walking through a farmer's market and looking at all the fresh foods available. The variety is both beautiful and intimidating for some home cooks. At farmer's markets there is an abundance of meats and vegetables many of which are new to people. Some of those I talk to are reluctant to cook without a detailed recipe. They simply don't know what to do with a new food or are afraid to venture out and try a new way to cook things. I can remember when my husband and I picked up our first order of beef that we purchased from a friend who raised her own cattle. We were handed several boxes of white freezer-paper-wrapped bricks of frozen meat. They were all different shapes and sizes, some of which were stamped with parts I had never heard of before. Laughing out loud, I asked my husband, "What's an arm roast?" It's fun to try new things. Let this section be a guide for you as you start your journey toward fresh food.

I want to teach you what I have learned about cooking, food, seasoning, and how to create delicious meals for your family that can be prepared with little effort. God created wondrous variety in our food. We should be able to mix and match different flavors to keep our appetites stimulated. To do this, I need to show you a little bit about how God designed our food.

I will walk you through what I've learned about animal foods: meat, bones, fats, dairy, eggs and organ meats. There is much confusion about how to properly prepare meats, fats, broths and organ meats. We will also discuss fresh milk, or raw milk, in detail. There are some guidelines you can follow to make sure your family is getting the best milk available. Eggs are an easy way to feed a large family. They are so versatile and can be prepared in many different ways. Fats are essential for energy and proper hormone development. Organ meats are highly prized for their mineral content. These animal foods are the backbone of our diets and give us the energy and fuel needed to get through the day.

When it comes to plants, I don't classify them the same way other people do. We will take a look at plant food groups: fruit (of the plant), stalks and leaves, roots and tubers, grains and legumes, and using flavor-potent herbs and spices. When I talk about fruits, this is where I lump all fruits together: apples, pumpkins, peaches, squash, tomatoes, peppers – anything that bears seed on the inside. Many of the same techniques can be used to coax flavor from the "fruit" of these plants. Stalks and leaves are not as flavorful but are wonderful sources of fiber and help to fill up an empty plate. I will show you how to pair these stalks and leaves with tasty animal fats and broths to truly bring out the flavor of these sorely neglected plant parts. Roots and tubers are bursting with flavor. In fact, they usually hold so much flavor that most people do not eat these by themselves. A little bit goes a long way, but boy, do they make our food taste good! Spices are extremely flavorful. Every region has basic combinations of spices that are used routinely in their foods. Usually these grow locally and are native to their area. They can help liven up a dull plate when you are bored with serving the same foods to your family. We will also talk about seeds: nuts, beans, legumes and grains. Grains and legumes are powerhouses of nutrients and fiber.

Then we will discuss salt and minerals. I believe these are an important part of our diet and must not be left out. Historically, salt and minerals have always been one product – natural sea salt. Unrefined sea salt is rich in minerals and does not need to be feared or used sparingly. There are also other great sources for minerals that are neglected.

Lastly, we will talk about natural sugars. Natural sugars are rich in minerals and enzymes. They are an important part of our diet and probably the most misused part of our food today.

NUTRITION FOR FAMILIES AND CHILDREN

So, what does God's design for nutrition look like? Take a look at the front cover of this book. Every food group is pictured. There are animal meats, bone broths, and tasty dips made from organ meats. There are fresh vegetables, fruits, and sauces with herbs and dry rubs for flavor. There are eggs, cheese, whole grains and legumes for snacks, and living food drinks and sauces. There's no need to come up with elaborate plans for feeding your family. God has made this very simple and tasty! Every food He has made is nourishing.

There are three macronutrients, or major nutrients: fats, protein, and carbohydrates. All of these are necessary for good health and no group should be omitted. Animal fats and proteins are nutrient dense and plant foods provide carbs for energy. A healthy diet includes a good mix of all three groups. In Deuteronomy 32, The Song of Moses, when the Lord lists all the foods He nourished the nation of Israel with, He lists a good mix of all three macronutrients: "...fruit of the fields... honey from the rock, oil, curds and milk... fattened lambs and goats, choice rams... the finest kernels of wheat, the foaming blood of the grape." The importance lies in the fact that God created these foods to nourish us, we just need to eat them as close to fresh and unprocessed as possible. There are basic food groups that every family should have access to in order to properly nourish themselves. These should be either raised by the family or bought locally from small farmers who have made a commitment to raise healthy animals and produce.

Eggs: Eggs are a complete food. Chickens are easily raised by families that don't have much space, and children can raise chickens without much help from adults. Chicken, duck, goose... any poultry egg will do. Poultry also has the added benefit of providing meat, manure for tall and prolific fruit trees, and free home and lawn insect control. Birds love to eat insects and that creates a wonderfully rich, dark yellow yolk full of nutrients. Eggs raised from healthy chickens can be eaten uncooked with no fear of pathogens.

Animals for meat: Any livestock such as cattle, goats, sheep, or hunted animals such as deer, elk, bison. There are too many to list here. These animals will be able to produce bones for broth, fat for frying, organ meats for minerals, and joints for gelatin and healing the gut. Don't forget muscle meats for steaks, ground meat, and jerky. Grazing animals are the easiest animals to raise. They have a docile, gentle nature. It also doesn't take more than two or three large grazing animals to feed an entire family for a year. They provide fur, leather, wool, and manure for rich garden soil. Wild caught seafood is a staple in some parts of the world, especially those near the sea. There is an extensive variety of seafood available in these areas, not limited to just fish. The bones of fish and many sea creatures make excellent fish stock, broth, and bisques.

Milk: Cattle, goats, and sheep provide the added benefit of supplying the family with fresh milk and dairy products. Fresh, unpasteurized milk is loaded with beneficial microflora that boost the digestive system and immune system. Fresh milk is easily absorbed without needing a lot of digestion. As fresh milk sours, it becomes sour cream, cream cheese, or clabber and the souring (or fermenting) process makes the milk even easier to digest. Butter, yogurt, and cheese are easily made at home. Ghee and some homemade cheeses are shelf-stable providing a way to store dairy for future use without the need for refrigeration.

Organ meats from poultry or grazing animals: Liver is a powerhouse for nutrients. It is packed with so many minerals and nutrients that it actually tastes "metallic," almost like a vitamin. This can be made milder by soaking a few hours in raw milk. The milk helps neutralize some of the metallic flavor of the meat. It's a meat vitamin! And even better, the minerals found in liver are easier for your body to digest.

Fresh fruits and vegetables: Fruits, vegetables, roots and tubers are great sources for carbohydrates and fiber. Plants are also the source of all herbs for flavoring our food. Salt by itself isn't enough. Cold-pressed oils such as olive, coconut, peanut, and avocado give us rich flavor and fuel for our bodies. Oils also help prevent dry skin and can be used to preserve other foods.

Grains and legumes: Whole grains such as wheat berries, oats, beans, lentils, nuts, corn, and rice all fall into this category. These are full of minerals and are also high in fiber.

Source of authentic sea salt: Non-processed sea salt can be found in two main forms – sun dried ocean water and dried up salt beds, such as the ones near Salt Lake City, Utah and the Dead Sea. Sea salt is an essential nutrient, is rich in minerals and helps naturally preserve food.

Living foods: If a family has access to the above categories, they will have all they need to create living foods and drinks such as fresh dairy products, kefir, or lacto-fermented vegetables. We will discuss these in detail in the section "Understanding Fresh Food."

FINDING OUR WAY BACK TO THE FARM AND KITCHEN

What's the best way for a family to switch to local, fresh foods? To most families, cooking everything from scratch seems like a daunting task. I agree. I have no intention of making everything from scratch. Making the switch is a journey, not a one-time goal. Good news! – it doesn't take much to start seeing improvements in your health and gut. Starting from when I first read *Nourishing Traditions* by Sally Fallon, it took our family four years to get to the point where we were buying fifty percent of our foods local or fresh, raw ingredients. That was many years ago and still, there is a box of cheese balls above the fridge, a can of hot cocoa mix on the counter, and way too much candy leftover from the holidays still lying around the house. We still go out to eat on occasion. Be practical about what your intentions are and give yourself room to make mistakes.

You will also need help from your spouse, whoever is living in your household. Be willing to compromise. When we first started drinking raw milk, I put chocolate syrup in it for my husband. It takes time to get used to the flavor. Fresh milk tastes richer, and now that we are used to the flavor we love it. Milk from the grocery store tastes like water. Life change happens slowly. It takes time and many different taste tests (like ten times or more) before some people will eat something new. Patience is key.

Before you get started, you will need:

A sense of adventure. When I began trying to make lacto-fermented pickles, my husband would not taste them but waited to see if the kids would eat them. I always tasted everything myself first, then waited a few days before serving to my husband. I think he was waiting to see if I lived.

An appreciation for farmers. To be exact, an appreciation for local farmers. In order for farmers to make a decent living, and in order for there to be a bright future for young farmers, we have to allow them to charge us for their hard work. You are paying someone for their hard work and labor. They planted the seeds and raised the vegetables. They pulled weeds. They raised the animals and cared for them. They fed chickens and cleaned out coops. They scrubbed water troughs and mended fences. If it is a value-added product, like baked bread or preserves, then there is even more labor involved. Pay them for their time.

An understanding of how government subsidizing has crippled food pricing. You cannot compare farmer's market prices to those at the grocery store. The quality of food at the farmer's market is superior, and the market is providing jobs for local people. The money from processed food is subsidized by tax dollars. Subsidized foods are priced artificially low. They are usually priced lower than anyone could produce the item for, even working at minimum wage. If farmer's market prices are too steep for you, find ways to get the most nutrient-dense foods for what you can afford. Sometimes you can get animal bones and liver for free. Use the whole vegetable or animal and keep waste to a minimum.

Okay, here's what I call the "Road to Fresh Food." It's a basic road map for families who don't know where to begin.

Keep in mind, it will probably take a year or more to get through the first four steps. Every family's journey is different. This is just a guideline.

1. Begin Cooking. This may sound a little obvious, but you would be surprised how many people have asked me how to eat healthy, only to find out they never cook at home. Begin cooking – you can always swap out store bought ingredients for fresh, local food later. The point is to get in the kitchen and start finding ways to make something tasty. Grill, smoke, marinate, fry and roast. If you're short on time, fill up a slow-cooker before leaving to go to work in the morning and return to a home-cooked meal waiting for you. Slow cookers are amazing!

2. Start drinking a probiotic cultured drink such as milk kefir, water kefir, or kombucha. These drinks are loaded with beneficial microflora that promote a healthy gut and boost the immune system. Some drinks can be purchased at grocery stores and others can be made at home. Check out the section called "Living Foods" for more details about these nourishing drinks and lacto-fermented pickles.

3. The next step is easy: Start using quality animal fats and oils. Butter, tallow (beef fat), lard (pork fat), schmaltz (chicken fat), ghee (clarified butter) and drippings saved from previous roasts are a few of our favorites. Ask around local butcher shops for beef fat and pork fat. Sometimes you can get these items for free if you call ahead of time. These are excellent for high heat frying as well. See the section on "Animal foods: Fats" on how to render fats. Peanut oil is another good choice for high heat cooking. Coconut and olive oil are perfect for salad dressings. We love to save the drippings and fat

from frying or roasting meats and use these for cooking vegetables. Your vegetables will vastly improve in flavor.

4. Decrease the amount of sugar in your food. Keep an eye on how much sugar and empty carbs your family is eating. Sodas, sweet tea, candy, pasta, white rice, dehydrated potatoes are all culprits. Watch for hidden sugar in things like spaghetti sauce and juice.

5. Find local farmers. Farmer's markets are the easiest place to find local farmers. Also look for food co-ops, CSA's or Community Supported Agriculture. In a CSA, you pay a monthly fee and pick up (or are delivered) a basket of farm fresh food weekly. Each basket differs according to what is being grown that season, and is a great way to get a variety of fresh food. Farm-shares are new and a great way to "own" a portion of a large animal and receive a portion of that animal's produce, such as milk or dairy products. Please visit the Farm-to-Consumer Legal Defense Fund website for more info on farm shares, co-ops and CSAs. Some great foods to look for are eggs, milk, beef, chicken, fresh fruit and veggies, and honey. If you live near the ocean, visit your local fish market. It's a great place to find fresh seafood.

6. Add variety to your food. If you've made it this far, you probably have some odd slices of beef stuck in the back of the freezer because you don't know how to cook them, lots of fresh and frozen veggies... and you're sick of eating the same ten meals. That's okay. It happens to everybody. We all get stuck in a cooking rut. Time for some inspiration! I love Taste of Home magazine because they feature meals and recipes from home cooks all over the nation. I always keep a few issues of their annual holiday magazine on the shelf. Allrecipes.com is another great resource. You can research recipes for different ethnic foods, new foods and flavors, and each recipe is rated by those who have tried to cook them.

Also, remember to follow the seasons in your cooking. Summer foods are lighter with more fresh fruit than winter foods. Winter foods are perfect for roasted meat, hearty chili and stew, and deep-fried potatoes.

7. Begin milling your own grains or buying whole grain flour that has been fresh-milled. It is important to eat whole grains, with the germ and bran. It is also important to eat bread that has not been made from bleached, refined flour. The rich oils and vitamins in the bran and germ go rancid quickly, and it is important to eat these from grains that are fresh milled.

8. Make or buy quality condiments. Homemade condiments are much healthier for your family. Over the years, I have learned that making condiments seems to be based on time available. However, some are very simple to make. Manufacturers are also meeting the demands of those who no longer which to purchase soy or canola in their condiments and sauces. Homemade relishes and chutneys are amazing and bursting with flavor. You can also use the opportunity to replace the soy and canola oils with healthy oils.

9. Preserving and storing food. Lacto-fermented foods such as homemade sodas, salsas, condiments and pickles are a fantastic source of living foods. They are also fun to make. When buying foods and whole vegetables from farmer's markets, you may notice that some items such as turnips and collard greens are huge! Turnips with greens (leaves) still attached can be 24" in length. Collard greens can grow even larger. You may want to start rinsing and freezing the leaves for later use. Dehydrating is also good for storing up and saving plant foods. I store bags of beans and dehydrated vegetables in the pantry and render fats, storing the fats in glass jars in the fridge. Raw vinegars are another way to store living foods.

Awareness and Transparency

When it comes to buying local food, especially meat, milk or eggs, one of the most important things you need to do is visit the farm before you start buying food. You need to see the animals with your own eyes. This seems daunting to someone who has never even seen a farm, but let me encourage you, it is easier than you think.

First, you should know that farms are very diverse. If you visit a hundred local farms, you will see a hundred different ways to do things. Doing things differently doesn't mean that it's wrong. Farmers are inventive. They find new ways to repurpose old items and structures. They have to; buying new materials all the time gets expensive. A working farm always has several projects going on at once. Enjoy the diversity of the different farms you visit.

Thankfully, there are some very basic clues you can look for as indicators of whether or not a farm is being managed well. These will not help you sort out excellent farms from mediocre farms, but it will help you spot farms that are truly managed poorly. There are a few things that decent farms will never have:

> *The smell of ammonia.* I'm not talking about the smell of poop, which every farm has. I'm talking about walking into or near an area that smells so bad of urine and ammonia that you cannot breathe. The smell of ammonia knocks you over. These animals are usually confined on dirt or concrete in an area that is too small for the animals to move around.

> *Small, permanent structures that do not move, where the animal spends its entire life.* No animal should be permanently confined to a small space with a concrete or bare dirt floor.

All animals need some sort of fresh grass or thick bedding and a place where they can walk away to poop and then return to clean, fresh bedding. Animals in permanent cages cannot get away from their own manure.

Nasty water. Obviously, there are animals that graze near ponds and such, but water troughs should at least look clean enough to drink from. Slime, sludge, worms and such should never be in the animals' water supply.

Let me tell you a few things we learned firsthand. When we first started buying local meat, I had no idea what healthy farm animals were supposed to look like. I doubted I would even be able to tell if the farm was a good one or not because I had never even been to a farm. But we had to start somewhere! We ended up buying beef from a lady advertising fresh, local beef with no hormones. We bought the meat right from the farm. As we drove down the driveway to a large two-story barn, we noticed the pasture on both sides of the driveway. Cows were munching in a field of grass on the right side and looked as healthy as we could tell from the car. They weren't skin and bones, they looked okay. We asked the lady as many questions as we could think of, and she happily answered them. She said she has grain fresh milled in town for her cows, just to supplement the finishing stage (last few weeks before they are butchered) and does not administer any growth hormones. She said she was giving medicine to one cow who had a hoof issue, but it was only temporary until the hoof healed, only a few more days or so. That was fine with me. I didn't mind a little medicine given to a cow who needs it. Good grief, I give medicine to my own children when they need it! We purchased several boxes of frozen meat and drove home. The meat was fantastic!

About a year later, we decided we wanted to raise our own

chickens for eggs. We found an advertisement posted on a bulletin board at the local farm store advertising baby chicks for sale. I made a phone call and spoke to the woman selling the chicks. She offered a fair price and gave us the address of her farm so we could come by and purchase them. We drove down the driveway of the farm and noticed a few peculiarities as we arrived. There were animals everywhere in cages, permanent cages. There were all kinds of animals; ducks, turkeys, chickens, goats, ...all caged with nothing but dirt underneath them. We did something we would never do now. We got out of the car and talked to her about the chickens. She led us to a barn where she had cages of chickens in various stages of growth. Some baby chicks, some only a few months old. Again, all dirt under the birds and all in permanent cages. It smelled bad. Really bad. She opened a cage and began handing my husband and I two-month old chickens. Fear gripped me as I realized the bird she handed me was covered in fleas. The bird she handed my husband was even worse. It had so many fleas that the fleas were crawling on its comb and all over its head, even near its eyes. When we mentioned the fleas, she promptly reached over and grabbed a spray bottle of some liquid and sprayed the chicken in the face. I looked at my husband and he looked at me with a look that said, "How fast can we get out of here?" We gave the birds back to the woman and left. When we got home, we dipped our shoes in chlorine, then put all of our clothes in the wash. Today, we would never even get out of the car at a farm like that.

Beyond the obvious, start reading books or visiting websites that talk about farm animal care. If your county has a 4H or FFA fair, visit and ask questions. Farm supply stores often have a rack of books on farm animal care. Be a well-informed consumer. Also, be aware of different farming practices. Be able to recognize the difference between a cattle operation that overcrowds their cattle versus a farm that practices mob-stocking and rotation. They might look the same from the road.

Buying fresh milk is little more complicated. There are a few things you should know before you begin. Is it legal to buy fresh, raw milk in your state? The Farm to Consumer Legal Defense Fund is a wonderful website dedicated to making sure that consumers have direct access to small farms, fresh milk and other nutrient-dense foods. You can find them at https://www.farmtoconsumer.org. They have information about herd shares and co-cops where consumers can purchase raw milk and a raw milk production handbook. The Campaign for Real Milk is another foundation that is dedicated to helping families find raw milk. They have an interactive state-by-state map with a review of raw milk laws. It can be found at https://www.realmilk.com. Their website answers many questions about raw milk such as raw milk safety, raw milk safe handling, and answers to many other questions. As of 2017, there are only eight states where raw milk sales are still illegal, but efforts are being made to amend or remove these restrictions.

ANIMAL FOODS

In defense of red meat and pork, I will quote this verse from the Bible because it's an eye opener!

> "Now the Spirit speaketh expressly, that in the latter times some shall depart from the faith, giving heed to seducing spirits, and doctrines of devils; speaking lies in hypocrisy; having their conscience seared with a hot iron; forbidding to marry, *and commanding to abstain from meats, which God hath created to be received with thanksgiving of them which believe and know the truth.* For every creature of God is good, and nothing to be refused, if it be received with thanksgiving: for it is sanctified by the word of

God and prayer." I Timothy 4:1-5 KJV (emphasis mine)

I love it! I can't tell you how many times I've been disappointed with the covers of magazines and posters talking about healthy food that proudly display only vegetables and fruit. Glossy covers, great photography... and only fruits and vegetables. Sometimes someone will be brave and include a small piece of chicken or slice of fresh fish on the cover, but red meat, beef or pork? Forget it!

Let's not forget this verse as well:

In Genesis 9:1-3, the Bible says, "Then God blessed Noah and his sons, saying to them, 'Be fruitful and increase in number and fill the earth. The fear and dread of you will fall upon all the beasts of the earth and all the birds of the air, upon every creature that moves along the ground, and upon all the fish of the sea; they are given into your hands. Everything that lives and moves will be food for you. Just as I gave you the green plants, I now give you everything.'"

Also, the Lord told Peter "Do not call anything impure that God has made clean" in Acts 10:6.

It's really important that we don't miss this: God has given us everything for food. With so many diet trends and agencies telling us to avoid animal foods: red meats, fats, whole milk, cream, eggs... it's easy to get confused and misled. I want to put this into perspective. When you avoid animal products, you are ignoring almost *half* of the foods God has given us. And you are ignoring the most nutrient-dense foods available. It's important to understand the difference between meat from grass-fed animals raised on small, local farms versus meat from animals raised in factory-like settings.

I want to note here what the Bible says about treating each other respectfully, even when we have different viewpoints about food. Romans 14 verses 1-4 says, "Accept him whose faith is weak, without passing judgment on disputable matters. One's man's faith allows him to eat everything, but another man, whose faith is weak, eats only vegetables. The man who eats everything must not look down upon him who does not, and the man who does not eat everything must not condemn the man who does, for God has accepted him. Who are you to judge someone else's servant? To his own master he stands or falls. And he will stand, for the Lord is able to make him stand." The argument about whether or not to eat meat is thousands of years old, so let's treat each other with kindness. For those who choose to eat meat, let's make sure we're eating meat from healthy animals raised on pasture-based local farms.

Animal products in the United States are underused. Typically, we eat the muscle meat and throw everything else away. The irony here is that muscle meats hold the least nutrition of the whole animal. The bones, fat and organs of an animal are nutrient dense. The trick is knowing how to use these in cooking so that you're getting the most benefit from these items. We'll talk about these in detail.

Meat

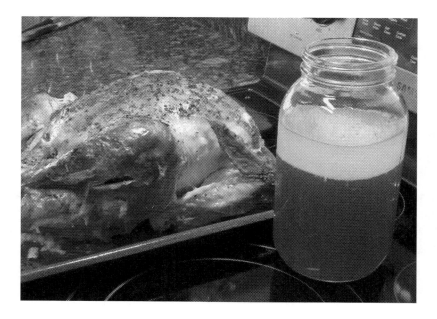

Let's start with muscle meats, just to discuss a few basics about keeping meat moist and tender. It's not that hard to sear a juicy red steak, but what about all those tough cuts of meat? To cook them properly, they can be slow-roasted until the tough tendons and cartilage melt into the juices and create outstanding flavor and tender meat. Muscle meat marbled with fat is the easiest to cook. It contains its own moisture. Water does not make meat moist – fat makes meat moist. When slow roasting or smoking meat, place the meat in the smoker fat side up. This allows the fat to slowly melt into the meat keeping it tender and juicy.

When roasting meat, the fat cooks out and melts into the juices surrounding the meat. I always save this fat whenever possible. This fat that cooks out of the meat is called "drippings" and makes an amazing gravy. I pour the hot drippings into canning jars and store them in the fridge. These jars of drippings are my go-to when I need to make a tasty gravy or add flavor to frozen veggies.

Meat by itself does not have much flavor, but it will absorb the flavor of the salt, herbs and spices around it. Salt brings out the natural flavor of meat. When coupled with a brine soak or marinade, the flavor of the meat triples. It has time to soak up the herbs and spices. What's even better is that soaking meat in a brine bath in the fridge buys you time. Brine simply means soaking the meat in heavily salted water. You can soak a whole chicken or pork shoulder in a brine bath for a day, two days or more and the salt prohibits bad bacteria growth. It doesn't kill bad bacteria, but it will slow it down. Poultry and pork work especially well with a brine bath.

Another great way to add flavor to muscle meats is smoke. It adds wonderful dimension to bacon, ham, large pieces of meat and roasts. Smoke from chips of pecan wood, apple, hickory and many other kinds of fruit and nut trees create rich flavor in meat. Don't have the time to smoke a large piece of meat? Authentic smoked sea salt or smoked paprika are great shortcuts for adding that rich, smoky flavor to meat cooked on the stove. They are powerful, though, so use sparingly. Smoked salt or smoked paprika, spices, and sometimes sugar can be combined to make a meat rub. Thoroughly coat the meat with the rub and let it sit in the fridge for several hours or a day and then cook the meat. Meat rubs with the right proportion of salt and sugar can also be used to "home cure" fresh meats like hams and bacon. This process is not equal to commercial curing, but will flavor the meat enough that it will be delicious. An excellent book for more details regarding curing and smoking is "Meat Smoking and Smokehouse Design" by Stanley, Adam and Robert Marianski.

Menu Planning for Less Waste

Menu planning is an art that has fallen away over time as we have grown ever more dependent on convenient foods. Menu planning for families is essential and reduces wasted food and unused leftovers. It's also not that difficult. It just requires about ten minutes a week to sit down and think through what is going to be prepared for the next seven days. Before you balk at the time it takes to sit down and plan meals, just think about how much time is wasted running to the grocery store to pick up a few last-minute items!

Menu planning looks at the meal being prepared for one day and makes sure the leftovers are incorporated into the next day's meal. For example, a roast chicken prepared on the first day can be sliced up and divided among the family. The chicken frame and any attached bits of leftover meat can be used to augment following meals. The second day, any leftover scraps can be pulled from the bones and used to make chicken pot pie. The bones can be used in a slow cooker to make chicken broth, then on the third day, the broth can be used to make egg drop soup. There is very little waste when each piece is maximized this way. Ground beef can be used to make tacos, then shepherd's pie over mashed potatoes. Leftover beef roasts can be chopped and put in chili or sliced for fajitas. Leftover pork chops can be used in spicy jambalaya or Latin pork and yellow rice. Just think, for every day you recycle leftovers, you are also saving cooking time! Typically, the meals that incorporate the leftovers are quicker and easier to prepare. After all, the meat is already cooked. You are just reheating it on the stovetop and adding some extra spices. To prevent having the same meat three days in a row, juggle two different types of meat. For example, roast a chicken the first day,

> then make pork chops the second day; chicken pot pie the
> third day, then spicy jambalaya with cooked pork on the
> fourth day, and so on.

Fast Food (30 minutes or less)

Seafood Dip

Seafood dip is one of those items that usually has a long list
of hard-to-pronounce ingredients. Good news! It's not difficult
to make yourself. I use a soft, creamy cheese base then add tiny
canned shrimp and bonito flakes for that rich seafood flavor.
Bonito flakes are light, paper thin shavings of dried fish. Usually
bonito flakes have a rich, slightly smoky flavor as well. They are
perfect for adding to dips and soups to add depth and dimension
to flavor. Cans of tiny shrimp can usually be found where cans
of tuna are sold. Bonito flakes can be found in the grocery store
next to soy sauce, in Asian markets, or online. If you cannot
find bonito flakes, you could use smoked paprika or smoked sea
salt to add that slightly smoky flavor.

2 cups ricotta cheese (or cream cheese – two 8 oz. pkgs. softened)

half stick or ¼ cup butter, softened (4 tbsp.)

10-15 medium cooked shrimp, diced (or 1 can tiny shrimp)

6 grams bonito flakes (or about 2 tbsp. crushed flakes)

Sprinkle of cayenne, paprika, onion, garlic, salt and lemon juice.

Mix all the ingredients together in a bowl. A light sprinkle of
lemon juice helps to balance the seafood flavors.

Variation: Smoked Salmon Dip

This is another easy, creamy dip that is high in protein. Follow the instructions above, only instead of adding shrimp and bonito flakes, use fresh cooked or canned salmon as the meat in the dip. Sprinkle with lemon juice if the dip tastes too "fishy." Add smoked paprika for a little smoky flavor.

How to cook Bacon

To cook bacon evenly, it needs to be cooked in bacon fat. It sounds almost scandalous to cook bacon in bacon fat, I know. But in order to cook a small, thin piece of meat that curls as it cooks, it requires "deep frying" in fat. Otherwise, you have burned patches on both sides with pockets of undercooked meat in the middle. I keep a jar in the cabinet where I pour the bacon fat and save it for future bacon frying later (this bacon fat is also *amazing* for frying potatoes!).

If you don't have any bacon fat saved up, you will need to find a tempered glass jar such as a Mason jar or canning jar. Better yet, you can look for a stainless steel can with a lid and filter specifically for saving bacon fat. Thrift stores might be another great place to look, considering saturated fats became unpopular decades ago. Most people have tossed out these very handy little cans for saving fats. You can also buy them online.

To build up a little jar of bacon fat, you will need to fry up 8-10 slices of bacon to get started. Place a frying pan on the stove and line the pan with a single layer of bacon covering the bottom of the pan and at least two layers of bacon along the sides. Without the bacon fat to cook this bacon in, you will have to cook it very slow allowing time for the fat to melt out of the bacon. You will see the fat begin to melt and a layer of oil begin to build in the bottom of the pan. Once you have this layer of oil in the bottom of the pan, then you can turn up the heat slightly and cook faster if you wish. I wouldn't turn it up past medium heat, though. If the bacon fat starts popping at you, it's too hot; turn the heat down. Turn the bacon over about 2-3 times during the cooking process to keep it from curling too much. The bacon along the bottom will cook first, beginning to bubble and brown. Once a piece of bacon begins to look like its browning, it's almost done. Set a plate next to the stove for the cooked bacon, lining the plate with a paper towel if you wish. As they begin to brown, move one piece of bacon at a time to the plate. The bacon will be crunchy as it cools. Take the bacon out of the pan before it turns dark brown. Once the bacon looks like it's "foaming," it will be well done. I usually remove the bacon before it starts foaming.

Once the bacon is cooked, turn off the heat and let the frying pan cool for about ten minutes. Get your jar ready with a funnel if desired. A metal, washable coffee filter makes a good strainer for catching bits of bacon, although it won't hurt anything if you end up with bits of bacon in the saved bacon fat. Pour the warm bacon fat through the strainer and into the jar. Put a lid on the jar and set it in a cabinet or on the counter. It does not need to be refrigerated. If you forget to pour the bacon fat into the jar and it cools and begins to solidify, it is still fine to save; just place the frying pan back on the burner for a minute or so until the fat begins to melt again.

Now that you have a jar of saved bacon fat, you can use this fat for the next batch of bacon. To cook the next batch of bacon, just spoon out about 2-3 tablespoons of bacon fat, then place the bacon in the bottom of the frying pan and cook as usual. By the way, cooking bacon is an excellent way to build seasoning on cast iron frying pans!

Cubed Steaks

1 cup of flour
1 tbsp. onion powder
2 tsp. salt

4-5 cubed steaks
1-2 cups of beef broth for making gravy
Additional spices such as garlic, thyme, or oregano

Start by mixing flour, onion powder and salt on a plate. Thoroughly coat both sides of the steak in the flour mixture. Save remaining flour for gravy. Melt lard, tallow, peanut oil or other oil for high-heat frying to ¼" deep. Heat the oil in the frying pan on medium heat. Gently place steaks in pan and cook for 3-7 minutes per side until flour has browned, or to your preference. Sprinkle steaks with additional onion, salt and spices such as garlic, thyme or oregano if desired.

Once steaks are cooked, pour off excess oil leaving several tablespoons in the pan for making gravy. Place a glass of water next to frying pan. Add 1-2 tablespoons of leftover flour mixture to oil in pan. Stir the flour and oil mixture in the pan over medium heat until flour has lightly browned. Once flour has browned, add the water to halt the browning process. Stir the gravy continually until water is thoroughly mixed in and begins to boil. See instructions in "Fats: Making Gravy" for more details. Once the water has boiled down to the right thickness, remove pan from heat and pour gravy into a serving dish.

Simple Steak, olive oil and salt

Choice cuts of steak have enough flavor on their own to be delicious. They don't need added spices and flavor, though that's perfectly fine if you choose to add them. Usually olive oil and sea salt are all that is needed to grill a fine steak. Steaks can be pan fried in a cast iron frying pan. Salt steaks and add a small amount of oil a few hours before cooking if time permits. Start at a higher heat at first to lock in the juices and then cook at medium heat until you have reached your cooking preference, rare, medium, well, etc...

Shrimp & Grits

The first time I tasted this dish, I had ordered it at the House of Blues in Orlando. I wasn't sure if I would like the combination, but then soon fell in love with it! This dish is how my family first began to eat grits. They wouldn't eat them before. Shrimp and grits is basically a corn grit "cake" covered in a rich, creamy, spicy sauce with fresh shrimp poured all over the grit cake. When I make this dish at home, I always add fresh halved cherry tomatoes and sneak in some other vegetables my family normally won't eat. The sauce is so rich and flavorful that I can usually get some diced yellow squash or zucchini in unnoticed.

2 tbsp. butter
30 shrimp, uncooked medium size
10-15 Halved cherry tomatoes
1 cup diced yellow squash, okra, bell pepper, fresh spinach or other vegetable of your choice (something that will cook quickly, about as much time as the shrimp)
½ cup heavy whipping cream
1 tsp. minced garlic
Sprinkle of cayenne, to taste
Sprinkle of salt
Cooked grits

Start by making a small pot of grits on the stove, about ½ to ¾ cup per person. Preheat the oven to 350 and oil or butter a muffin baking sheet. When the grits are fully cooked, pour them into muffin cups, filling each muffin cup to the top. Bake for 15-20 minutes or until the tops are slightly browned and the grit cakes are dry around the edges.

While they are baking, place the butter into a frying pan, melting the butter. Add fresh or frozen uncooked shrimp and cook on medium heat. Add the vegetables to the shrimp and cook together until the shrimp are cooked (they will turn pink and curl). Turn the heat down to low, and add the cream, garlic and spices. Stir until all the flavors have combined well, a minute or two, then remove from the heat.

Place one or two grit cakes top-side down in a bowl and ladle the shrimp, vegetables and sauce over the grit cakes. Serve while hot. If you don't like the taste of grits, this dish is also tasty served over a slab of cornbread.

Slow Food (hours)

Slow Cooker Pot Roast

1 beef roast
3-4 large carrots
4-6 small to medium size potatoes
2 small onions
1 tsp. sea salt
Your favorite meat rub or oregano, basil and thyme

The trick to making a good pot roast is to sear the roast before cooking it. Add a tablespoon of oil to a frying pan and heat the oil to medium. Using tongs, hold each side of the roast in the frying pan until each side is browned. The roast will still be raw on the inside. Transfer roast to slow cooker lined with potatoes and carrots. Liberally top roast with minced onions and salt. To transform this roast from delicious to spectacular, add a generous coating of your favorite meat rub, especially one that has a little smoked sea salt or smoked paprika. We prefer rubs that are labelled "no MSG."

To make a pot roast that has a gravy instead of clear juice, mix 1/3 cup of flour with 1 cup of beef broth (or water with a little salt and spices such as garlic and thyme) in a small bowl. Pour this mixture over the roast. This will run down into the slow cooker and melt into the juices from the roast and create a fabulous gravy. Cook on high for 8 hours or until meat is fork tender.

Roast Chicken

I like to roast a whole chicken in the oven in oven roasting bags. This collects all the juices from the chicken and allows me to save all the drippings for broth. The bags also help keep the meat moist. Rinse and place the chicken on a large platter or plate. If the chicken was purchased from a store, remove any giblets or bags from the inside (see Chicken Pate' for a great recipe using chicken liver; it's a dip made from butter, chicken broth, and chicken liver – very tasty!). Sprinkle the chicken liberally with sea salt and your favorite combination of spices, such as lemon and minced garlic.

Pour about 1 tablespoon of olive oil into the roasting bag and spread the oil around in the bag (I roll up the bag, forcing the oil into all the corners of the bag) then open the bag and place the chicken inside. Place the chicken in the bag breast side up into a deep roasting pan, at least 1 ½" deep. The bag will collect a lot of juices from the meat as it cooks. Add any veggies you desire, such as celery, onions or carrots. Tie the bag in a knot to seal it. Cut a 1" hole in the top of the bag above the chicken, then place in the oven.

Roast the chicken at 350 for 1 ½ hours or until juices run clear. When the chicken is done, allow to cool for ten minutes. To collect the juices for broth, carefully cut open the bag and lift the chicken out of the roasting pan. Lift the bag out of the pan, being careful not to spill the juices. Remove any large chunks of cooked vegetables with tongs, then pour roasting pan contents through a strainer into a large bowl. All of this juice is chicken drippings and makes a wonderful broth, soup or gravy! Pour the drippings into a jar with a lid and store in the fridge for up to a month.

There are endless varieties of meat rubs and spices that add wonderful flavor to a roast chicken. If you plan to save the juices for broth, though, I would not add any rubs that contain sugar. Chicken broth does not taste right when it's sweet.

Variation: Roast Rooster!

We've found that roosters are best cooked in a slow cooker. The meat is a little tougher, but they generally have huge legs and tasty drumsticks. Place the rooster, cleaned and rinsed, in the slow cooker breast side up on top of a thick layer of onions, celery, and carrots. Liberally salt the rooster and sprinkle with lemon juice. Cook for about 3 hours on high, or 6-7 hours on low. If you have a particularly large rooster, it may need more cooking time. If your rooster will not fit in the slow cooker, cut up into pieces, separating the legs and thighs from the frame. Reduce the cooking time to 2 ½ hours on high or 5-6 hours on low. Cook until juices run clear. Remember to save the juices from your farm-fresh rooster! They make delicious, rich chicken drippings and gravy.

Easy Chicken Pot Pie

Roast chicken leftovers make a wonderful chicken pot pie. I have the children pick all the leftover meat from the chicken frame, and we turn those bits of meat into a delicious meal.

Filling:
2 tbsp. butter
1 small onion diced
1 tbsp. flour
½ tsp. sea salt
1 cup chicken broth
1 cup peas
1 cup sliced carrots
½ cup sliced celery, spinach, or other vegetable
1 cup heavy whipping cream

Chicken meat pieces from leftover roast chicken frame, about
½ - 2 cups

Melt butter in frying pan. Add fresh onions; heat in butter
until softened and clear. Add salt and flour and stir until
thoroughly mixed. Lightly brown flour for 1-2 minutes, then
add about 1 cup chicken broth. Stir until thoroughly mixed. Add
peas, carrot slices and other vegetables and cook until tender.
Once vegetables are tender, add cream and cooked chicken.
Stir to thoroughly incorporate the vegetables and meat into
the sauce. Add more broth if needed to maintain the amount
of sauce in the frying pan. There should be plenty of sauce to
cover the vegetables and meat. Once thoroughly mixed, remove
from heat. Pour chicken mixture into a deep pie baking dish.

Pie Crust: 1 cup flour, ½ tsp. sea salt, 4 tbsp. butter softened

Mix the flour and salt together in a small bowl. Add softened
butter and stir with a fork, pressing into flour and mixing until
you have a crumbly, dry dough. The dough should stick together
when you press on it with the fork, but should break apart and
crumble as you stir it with the fork. Don't add water to this dough.
The flour must bake in the butter to become crunchy. Adding
water to flour creates chewy dumplings; not what we want for a
pie crust. If the dough is too dry, add a little more softened butter.
If too sticky, add a little more flour. Sprinkle these crumbles onto
the chicken filling until they completely cover the filling. Bake at
350 for about 10 minutes or until crust has browned.

Really Slow Food (days)

Smoked Pork Butt/Shoulder *Chris Hambelton*

Thaw one or two Boston butts, between 5 and 8 pounds
each. Brine them for 24-48 hours, depending on how much time

you have. To brine the pork, in a clean plastic bowl or dish pan, cover the pork with water so it is mostly submerged. Add a cup of sea salt or pickling salt spread evenly across the entire pan. It's okay if it rests on the meat that is above the surface of the water. Cover and place in the fridge for the allotted time. The nice thing about brining is that you can brine while waiting for the meat to defrost, if needed, by placing a frozen Boston butt in the brine solution.

After the brining is complete, drain off all of the water and then coat generously with your favorite dry-rub. I prefer flavor notes of smoky sweet rubs and apple wood. Make sure you buy quality rubs, no wheat additives or MSG. Once coated with the rub, place covered back in the fridge for up to 12hrs. In a pinch, I have gone straight to the smoker after applying the rub.

Place the prepped meat on the smoking rack, no need to use foil or a pan. Make sure the fat layer is on top. You want the fat to melt into the meat as it cooks. I prefer an electric smoker. Set the temp to 225 F, and add wood chips to the appropriate area (see smoker owner's manual), and set for 18 hours. Time tips: if you're having the pork for lunch, start the pork at 4pm the day before. If it's for dinner, start the smoker at 10pm.

Keep an eye on the internal temperature. Many smokers have temp probes that you can leave in the duration of cooking. Depending on humidity, altitude, and nuances of your smoker cooking times may vary. If it's not cooking fast enough, feel free to adjust temp up to 250 F. This is where you can get creative and use your culinary skills to perfect the process. An internal temperature of 195F makes for the most tender meat. Be careful not to go over 195F, that's the sweet spot...

Remove meat from the smoker and immediately wrap or cover tightly in foil. The meat needs to rest for about an hour. This helps improve the flavor and seal in juices. You are free to pull the pork at this point but I prefer to serve it whole. Set up a large fork and a knife and allow your guests to gauge the amount of bark (the smoked outside), remaining fat, and meat tenderness they prefer. Place on a bun or straight onto the plate and add your favorite sauce if desired, but remember, this meat is good enough, so don't hide your hard work with a bunch of sauce.

Fats

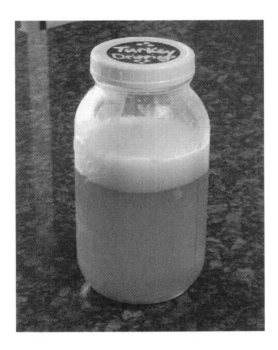

Most people don't realize that our bodies need animal fats in order to properly make hormones. Hormones regulate nearly everything in our bodies. Insulin is also a hormone, needed to process sugar. We need healthy animal fats in order to process sugar! Sugar consumption has skyrocketed in the last fifty years. Our consumption of animal fats has plummeted in the same amount of time. We are told to avoid the healthy animal fats our bodies need in order to be able to cope with all that sugar. It's a recipe for disaster.

Don't be afraid of quality animal fats. There are many ways

to get quality animal fats into your diet. The easiest way is to stop throwing them out! Animal fats can be saved from the drippings (or juices) that melt out of a chicken as it is roasting. Save these juices and keep them for cooking vegetables and making gravies. Stop trimming the fat off of steaks and roasts. Place roasts fat side up in the roasting pan so that the fat melts into the meat and keeps the meat moist while roasting. Use these high-quality fats to replace highly refined soy and canola oils.

Olive oils and coconut oils are excellent fats for salad dressings and medium temperature cooking, but for high-heat frying, nothing compares to rendered beef fat, called tallow.

Rendering animal fat

Rendering animal fats is an easy process. "Rendering" is simply melting the animal fat and saving the liquid fat in glass jars or containers for later. You need a large pot and a sharp knife. Start by slicing the fat into thin slices, about ¼" inch thick. Then cross-cut these thin slices into small cubes of fat about 1" to ½" in diameter. Place all the diced fat into a large pot and begin heating the pot on medium heat. Once you see fat melting on the bottom of the pan, begin stirring the diced fat occasionally. If the fat starts popping and bubbling, it's too hot. Turn the heat down. After about 15 minutes, you will notice a lot of golden yellow liquid building up in the bottom of the pot. Keep stirring until all the fat turns transparent.

Once all the fat is transparent and no longer opaque or white, you can begin to ladle the golden liquid tallow into jars. Keep the heat on and continue to ladle the liquid into jars until there is nothing left but browned pieces of fat leftover. These are called "cracklins" and are edible if you wish to eat them. They are great salted and sprinkled on top of salads. Usually, we only eat them salted if they are crunchy. If not, our dog loves a few pieces of cracklins on his dog food, and the beef fat keeps his skin healthy and his coat shinning.

Roast Tallow

Another, quicker option for rendering tallow is roasting it in the oven. It seems to melt faster, but also lends a stronger "roasted beef" flavor to the tallow. Cut the fat into small cubes, as small as you can. Then place the diced fat into a deep dish roasting pan. Bake at 300 until plenty of liquid golden fat has melted out of the fat.

Fried Potatoes in Tallow

Since you've worked so hard to render all this golden tallow, be sure to use it! Potatoes rise to new heights in flavor when fried in tallow. Dice potatoes and melt 2-3 tablespoons or more of tallow into a frying pan. Fry the potatoes on medium heat until crispy and golden brown. Sprinkle with sea salt and pepper or onion. Enjoy!

Making Gravy

Few things are as delicious as gravy, and – contrary to popular belief – gravy is not bad for you. Once you understand that healthy animal fats are not bad for your body, you will never have to eat dry meat again! The animal fats in gravy provide energy, lubricate the esophagus so lumps of meat and rice don't get stuck in the throat, and they make tough meat taste better. It's also easy to make once you understand the basic process.

Gravy has three basic steps. It's important to understand these steps because performing them out of order results in gooey, lumpy gravy. Or soupy flour. There are three ingredients to gravy: oil, flour, and broth. Memorize them in that order, because that's the order in which you add the ingredients. Here are the three basic steps: melt the oil, brown the flour in the oil, then add a glass of broth to halt the flour browning process.

Almost any oil or animal fat can be used to make gravy. Usually, the drippings or fat from the meat that was just roasted or fried works well. For example, the fat that rises to the top of turkey drippings is wonderful for making turkey gravy. Since water from the meat will mix with the fat into the drippings, I pour the drippings into a glass canning jar and let it sit for a few moments so the fat rises to the top of the jar. Then I spoon the liquid fat off the top for making gravy. The drippings from a beef roast also works well for making a beef gravy. One of my favorite gravies to use in a pinch, or for making extra gravy for leftovers, is butter gravy. It's simple, easy, delicately flavored and goes with almost anything.

Let's look at the steps of gravy-making in detail. We'll take a simple butter gravy for example.

First: Get a full glass of broth ready (about 1-2 cups) and set it next to a large frying pan. You'll need the broth ready at the right time to stop the flour from burning. Now melt the butter (or whatever animal fat from drippings you want to use) in the frying pan. Heat your oil in the frying pan on medium heat. About a fourth of cup of oil or butter should be enough for a half pan of gravy.

Second: When it's melted, add about three tablespoons of flour. Now here comes the important part: do *not* add any broth until the flour begins to brown on the bottom. This will take a minute or two. Stir the flour in the oil thoroughly to make sure all the flour is covered in oil. This will help prevent lumps later on. While you're waiting for the flour to brown, you can liberally sprinkle the flour with powdered onion, salt and pepper. Once the flour begins to brown, you will smell a noticeable difference in the flour. It will smell toasted, not like raw flour or dough. Once the flour is browned and the onion and salt are added, it should start smelling really good! The flour should be light to medium-colored brown, about the color of caramel.

Third: Halt the browning process by adding a full glass of broth. Don't panic if it looks lumpy at first, just keep stirring the gravy as it begins to boil. Once you have added the broth, you are done browning the flour. You are now boiling the gravy. Do not add any more flour after this step.

You can relax now, because it is impossible to burn the gravy at this point. You are now boiling off the water in the gravy until you get the right amount of water and thickness that you are looking for. If the gravy gets too thick, you can add more broth or water and boil it again until you get the thickness of gravy that you want. You can test this by dipping a spoon into the gravy and lifting it back up. Does the gravy look watery, or has it begun to thicken? Keep boiling it until it looks right.

While you are waiting for the water to boil down to the right thickness, get a clean spoon and taste the gravy. Does it need salt? More onion? You can add more drippings to increase the flavor if it needs more flavor. Try to make sure the flavor of the broth matches the flavors of the gravy. For example, broth from chicken roasted in garlic will go fine with beef roasted in garlic. Sugar glazed ham broth added to beef gravy... not so much. If it's too salty, don't add flour. Add a little more water to thin it and resolve next time not to add too much salt. If it's too thick, add more water to thin the gravy. Once the gravy is the right thickness and it tastes good, you are done! Serve immediately.

What about those who are gluten intolerant? Did you know that a very simple, clear gravy can be made by following all of the steps above and simply omitting the flour? The result is similar to au jus, or the clear gravy that comes with a French dip sandwich. The key is to start with a rich animal fat, then add lots of flavor; onion, salt and spices. I like to add whatever I used to flavor the meat, anything you would put in chicken or beef broth. Don't add sugar or sweet rubs! It won't taste right. When people taste gravy or au jus, they expect salty and savory, not sweet. Add broth slowly until you get the right intensity of flavor.

Bone Broth

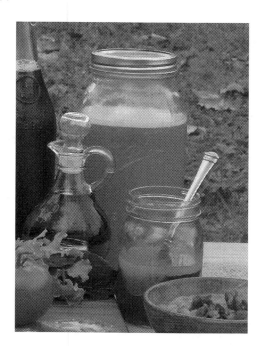

Bone broth is essentially broth made from the bones of beef, chicken, or fish. It's the old-fashioned way of cooking stock by simmering the bones with vegetables, spices and salt until the bones are soft and the cartilage is dissolved. A spoonful of acid such as apple cider vinegar or lemon juice helps the minerals in the bones dissolve into the broth. Think marrow bones, joints and bones that have cartilage attached are perfect for a rich, flavorful broth. Stock made this way with dissolved cartilage is full of gelatin that helps heal the gut and is rich in minerals.

The Big Three – Onions, Carrots, and Celery

A delicious broth can be created from the bones of grazing animals such as beef, and from poultry. Thick marrow bones and bones with cartilage attached are best but other bones work as well. Onions, carrots, and celery are the staple for any bone broth. All three are highly aromatic and bursting with flavor. Combined with a generous amount of sea salt, this type of homemade broth is superior in flavor and nutrition to any store-bought broth.

Preheat the oven to 350F. Arrange the bones along with a generous supply of carrots, celery, and onions on a large baking sheet. Don't cut the vegetables into small pieces. Keep them in large enough pieces that can be removed later using tongs. Brown the bones and vegetables in the oven for about 15-20 minutes. It is not necessary to cook them all the way through. Browning the bones first adds a richer, deeper flavor.

Note: For additional depth of flavor, bone broth can be made with wine drizzled over the bones and vegetables prior to browning. Red wine is usually paired with beef bones, and white wine with pork and poultry bones.

While the bones are in the oven, set a large pot on the stove and fill half way with water, or enough to cover the bones and vegetables. Put all of the bones and vegetables, along with juices that are on the baking sheet, into the pot and bring to a boil. Add a generous amount of sea salt, and if desired, 10-15 peppercorns. Add 1-2 tablespoons lemon juice or apple cider vinegar to aid as an acid, unless you drizzled the bones with wine (which acts as an acid). Once boiling, reduce heat to simmer, cover, and let cook for a minimum of 4 hours. The longer it simmers, the richer the flavor and more of the minerals and cartilage dissolve into the broth. This broth can simmer for 12 hours or more until the bones become pliable and can be easily indented with a utensil.

When the broth is done, taste the broth. If more salt is needed, add more salt to taste. Use tongs to remove the bones and vegetables. Ladle broth into canning jars and store in the refrigerator. The vegetables will be full of flavor and are excellent used in a casserole or stuffing. Bones that still contain marrow can be scooped out; use this cooked marrow as you would butter, or on toast in the recipe below. Roast bone marrow is also a rich and nutrient dense baby food for infants.

Note, a properly made broth will gel with fat on the top and will recombine upon reheating and stirring. Do not discard the top layer, it is highly flavorful and nutritious. The gelatin in this type of broth is nutrient dense and helps heal and seal the gut lining. Store in the fridge for 4-6 weeks.

Slow cooker bone broth

Line the slow cooker bottom and sides with carrots, celery and onions. Place bones in the center of the slow cooker (brown in oven as described previously if time permits). Fill the slow cooker with just enough water to cover the bones and vegetables. Add a generous amount of sea salt, and if desired, 10-15 peppercorns. Add 1-2 tablespoons lemon juice or apple cider vinegar to aid as an acid. Cover and cook on high for 10-12 hours. Once broth is done, taste broth. Add more salt if desired. Remove bones and vegetables using tongs and ladle into jars. Store in the fridge.

Roast Poultry Drippings (See Roast Chicken)

Salted Marrow on Toast

Believe it or not, roast marrow is delicious! It tastes like oil from a savory pot roast. It is very rich, so a little bit goes a long way. Save the bones with marrow (large open circles filled with fat inside the bone) from bone broths and roasts. Don't throw it away! Roasted bone marrow is nutrient dense and loaded with healthy fats. It is best served on something crunchy, like toast or French bread. I like to serve roasted bone marrow spread thinly on toast, lightly salted and sprinkled with crumbled bacon. Roasted marrow is also a great first food for babies.

How to Replace Cream of Chicken Soup in Recipes

I often use recipes that call for a can of cream of chicken soup. To replace a can of cream of chicken soup in a recipe, I use about ½ cup of heavy whipping cream or sour cream and about ½ cup of roast chicken drippings. The drippings should be salty enough to replace the salt in the can of soup. If not, add a little extra sea salt and some seasonings, such as celery or paprika, to add a flavor boost.

Cream of Mushroom Soup

I replace this ingredient with a healthy scoopful of sour cream, or about a ½ cup of heavy whipping cream and fresh or dried mushrooms. Add plenty of sea salt and some seasonings, such as diced or dried celery, paprika, or onion to add a flavor boost.

Liver

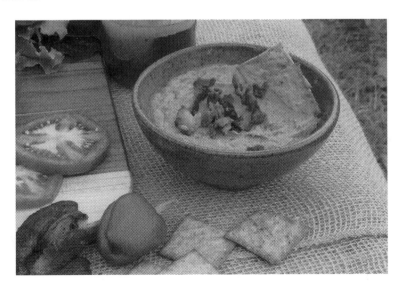

Soaking and Using Liver

Liver is sorely underutilized in American culture today. People are often turned off by liver because of its strong taste. This can be reduced by soaking the liver meat in raw milk for one to two hours at room temperature. Soak in a small dish with just enough milk to cover the meat. Raw milk is essential because it has active enzymes that help reduce the metallic taste and significantly improve the flavor of the meat. This little trick can be used for almost any kind of animal liver. It is worth mentioning here that the strong flavor of liver comes from the high content of minerals and vitamins. These nutrients are already in "meat" or animal form, which is easily absorbed by the human body. Radiant Life Company lists some of these reasons to enjoy liver from grass-fed beef:

- An excellent source of high-quality protein
- Contains all of the fat-soluble vitamins A, D, E and K
- Our most concentrated source of vitamin A, which is rapidly depleted during periods of stress, as well as by consuming a low-fat diet
- All of the B vitamins in abundance, particularly vitamin B12
- One of our best sources of natural folate
- A highly usable form of iron
- Trace elements such as copper, zinc, and chromium; liver is our best source of copper
- CoQ10, a nutrient that is especially important for cardiovascular function
- A good source of purines, nitrogen-containing compounds that serve as precursors for DNA and RNA

*Source: Radiant Life Desiccated Liver Capsules; blog.radiantlifecatalog.com

If liver is still not for you, powdered liver capsules are available at Radiant Life Company. My family doesn't like the taste of liver so we don't eat it as a meal, but instead we hide it in other spicy, flavorful foods. Liver that has been soaked, cooked, and finely diced can be added to meatballs, chili, taco meat, homemade sausage... the list goes on.

Potatoes with Bacon and Liver Crumble

Pre-soak a small piece of liver, 3-4 inches wide, in raw milk for 1-2 hours. Rinse liver and pat dry. In a small frying pan, fry 3-4 slices of bacon and liver in one tablespoon of butter. Sprinkle liver liberally with onion powder and cook about 5 minutes on medium heat, until cooked through. Dice cooked liver into very small pieces and crumble bacon. Chop potatoes into cubes and fry in a pan using butter or tallow. Add salt to the potatoes to taste. Once browned, add bacon and liver crumble (and the bacon fat from the frying pan) to the potatoes. Be sure to use plenty of onion as diced onion or onion powder help balance the liver flavor. Serve as a side dish.

Chicken Paté

Would you be more interested in trying paté if I told you it is primarily butter? That's right! This recipe is mostly butter, chicken broth, and mild chicken liver cooked into a thick paste. Tastes just like chicken soup. I never tasted chicken paté until I tried to make it at home. Once I saw how simple it was, we've been making it at home ever since.

Melt a half stick of butter in a small pot. Add 1-2 chicken livers and cook until meat is cooked through. You can take the liver out and slice on a plate to check for doneness. Add ½ cup of roast chicken drippings and heat the drippings until melted. Use a stick blender or food processor to puree the butter and liver mixture into a smooth, creamy consistency. Taste the mixture and add more salt if necessary. Pour into a small dish and keep covered in the fridge. This paté is excellent served cold with toast or crackers. Keeps about one week in the fridge.

Dairy

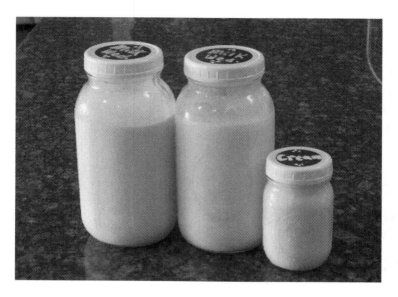

I once read in a cookbook published prior to 1960 that children should drink a quart of milk a day. I remember thinking at the time that was a lot of milk. A quart a day for each child! I would have to buy several gallons of milk a week just to feed the children. The average cow produces two gallons of milk a day. Dairy cows produce six gallons a day or more. It got me wondering about how our culture has turned its back on the dairy cow. Dairy cows were once the backbone of the family homestead. I can see why! With a little herd of five or six cows, a family could have gallons of fresh milk, every dairy product imaginable and a freezer full of beef. Talk about blessed! I can also see how children growing up with a family dairy cow would be blessed with lots of nutritious milk to drink for strong bones and healthy teeth; and if the milk is fresh and unpasteurized, lots of probiotics for the gut. I have a hard time believing any recommendations that we should reduce our dairy intake when these amazing grazing animals have been supporting family homesteads for thousands of years.

Fresh, unpasteurized milk is a versatile and nutrient-dense food. Raw milk is full of beneficial microflora. The calcium and minerals in raw milk are easily absorbed due to the enzymes naturally present in fresh milk. It is also full of healthy fats. Raw milk is able to be converted into many other dairy products by following multiple techniques. It can be made into tasty foods such as butter, buttermilk, cheese, ice cream, and all of the resulting dairy products made from raw milk will also contain the beneficial microflora. Fermenting, or souring, the milk into foods such as sour cream and kefir multiplies the probiotic microflora content and yields an acidic dairy product with a much lower pH, resisting pathogens.

Raw milk is highly nutritious and also highly disputed. Ron Schmid, ND, the author of The Untold Story of Milk, gives various examples of the risks and benefits of consuming raw milk. Schmid states, "Because much of the modern and historical debate about raw versus pasteurized milk involves issues of safety in relation to infectious disease, it is important to take a look at the current paradigm, the belief that germs cause illness. Those who maintain that illnesses commonly associated with certain germs are caused simply by exposure to those germs will view raw milk as a threat and a danger. But for those who believe that illnesses are caused by a failure of the immune system to adequately cope with infectious agents, the issue shifts and focuses instead on the building of powerful immunity, mainly through nutritious food. The basic choice that lies before

"The basic choice that lies before us is whether to choose foods that are nutrient-dense, or that have been rendered sterile."

us is whether to choose foods that are nutrient-dense, or that have been rendered sterile."

As mentioned before, there are some questions to consider before purchasing raw milk. Is it legal to buy raw milk in your state? The Farm to Consumer Legal Defense Fund is a wonderful website dedicated to making sure that consumers have direct access to small farms, fresh milk and other nutrient-dense foods. You can find state-by-state information about raw milk laws at https://www.farmtoconsumer.org. They also have information about herd shares and co-ops where consumers can purchase raw milk and a raw milk production handbook. The Campaign for Real Milk is another foundation that is dedicated to helping families find raw milk. They have an interactive state-by-state map with a review of raw milk laws. It can be found at https://www.realmilk.com. Their website answers many questions about raw milk such as raw milk safety, raw milk safe handling, and answers to many other questions. As of 2017, there are only eight states where raw milk sales are still illegal, but efforts are being made to amend or remove these restrictions. Ways to obtain raw milk are increasing, however, this does not mean that consumers can let their guard down. As with any food source (from FDA approved food to farmer's markets) there are opportunities to contaminate or deplete nutritional values. A Campaign for Real Milk, a project of the Weston Price Foundation, is an amazing resource to dig deeper into safety, access, and things to look for when purchasing raw milk. An informed consumer and transparency will help drive quality and safety in the food industry.

There are two different ways to milk a cow, by hand or by milking machine. Hand milking has an advantage when it comes to detecting mastitis in dairy animals because you can feel the clumps while milking even before a fine strainer will catch them (If a farmer is not hand milking, inexpensive equipment can be purchased online to detect mastitis). Mastitis is an infection from a clogged milk duct or a result of not being milked regularly. Don't drink this milk until the infection clears; let the milk fall onto the ground for over a week to allow for clearing of obvious signs of mastitis – some of which are clumps in the milk and pink-tinged milk. Mastitis can also be easily detected by letting the milk settle in a clear glass jar overnight in the fridge. As long as the milk is not homogenized, the cream will rise to the top overnight, and milk from a cow with mastitis will develop a pink line right between the milk and cream line. Unfortunately, the homogenization process covers up the ability to visually see mastitis symptoms in milk. The cream from goat's milk does not easily rise to the top like cow's milk does, but goats rarely ever get mastitis. It is also worth mentioning here that mastitis is easily corrected on small farms without medicine or antibiotics by simply adjusting the cow's milking schedule to make sure the cow's udder is milked frequently and completely at each milking. With correct milking technique, the symptoms will disappear within a few days.

Don't be afraid to ask questions at farmer's markets. This is where you need to get to know your farmer and build a relationship built on trust and transparency. The Raw Milk Institute (RAWMI) has published common standards and guidelines for what clean raw milk looks like and guidelines for testing raw milk. They have information for consumers, legislators, regulators, and farmers. They have information regarding education, training and listed farms that have registered with RAWMI and meet their common standards guidelines. Unfortunately, testing is not available or affordable in many areas for small farmers. I calculated the cost to get milk tested from one cow and it would cost around $140 a week. Yikes! The best defense is to talk to your farmers, go visit the farm, ask good questions, and be vigilant for shortcuts.

If raw milk isn't for you

If you don't feel comfortable buying raw milk, you have many options available to get living foods into your diet. Try experimenting with some of these foods. There is an entire chapter on Living Foods in Section Three, Understanding Your Food, where we will discuss how to make each food in detail.

Lacto-fermented vegetables: A method of making pickles and chutneys with either salt or whey before vinegar became the primary commercial way to make pickles. These are naturally fermented and tart, and they contain many probiotic and beneficial bacteria. They can be made dairy-free.

Water kefir: A homemade "soda" that can be made from any juice or fresh fruit. The kefir grains are similar to milk kefir grains, but thrive on natural sugars. They convert sugar into a mild vinegary-tart drink. They can be sweetened afterwards by adding more juice. By using air lock lids, you can create the same amount of carbonation as store-bought sodas. Grape juice produces a homemade soda that tastes exactly like sparkling grape juice. Some tasty options are strawberry soda, apple cinnamon soda, grape soda, pineapple ginger, etc. They have a wide variety of beneficial bacteria and yeasts. I think these drinks are the most mild and easiest for families new to living foods. They are more mild than kombucha and they are also dairy-free.

Kombucha: Stronger than water kefir, most kombucha takes a little getting used to. Sweet-tart and fizzy, kombucha is carbonated and full of beneficial bacteria, especially lactobacillus coagulans, the primary ingredient in Digestive

Advantage, a probiotic gummy. One benefit, however, is that kombucha can be purchased at most Publix and Target stores in the produce section. If they are too strong for you, they can also be mixed with juice to dilute the tart flavor. You can buy kombucha in many different flavors, but my personal favorite is GT's Strawberry Kombucha.

Milk kefir: Milk kefir grains are wonderful to work with and make a thin yogurt-like drink, but without all the fuss. Milk kefir also has a wide variety of beneficial bacteria and yeasts, more so than water kefir. If you don't want raw milk, start with pasteurized milk from grass-fed cows and add the kefir grains. After culturing, pour off the kefir, saving the grains to be used again. You can add fruit and flavors to your kefir to make all kinds of tasty options.

Yogurt: Yogurt is a great living food, but if buying commercially prepared yogurt, try to find a yogurt that is full-fat and contains at least several different strains of beneficial bacteria. These should be listed on the label. The temptation with yogurt is to buy the super-sweetened varieties with cookies and chocolate that are more like a dessert than yogurt. Just keep an eye on how much sugar you're eating.

Milking Basics (Just so Ya' Know)

I've included this basic information about how to milk a cow because families need to know this information if they are going to purchase fresh, raw milk. It's important to have a basic understanding of the process. So in a nutshell, here's the basic process:

First, start with a friendly cow. This may seem obvious but it is really important, especially for those who plan to hand milk their cows. Will the cow eat a treat out of your hand? Can you walk up to her and scratch her back? Will she let you rub her belly and touch her udder without kicking you? She needs to be friendly and used to human hands rubbing her belly. Dairy cows are not pets but they need to be comfortable with your touch.

Once you have a friendly cow, you need to get her to a place where you can milk her. Lead her onto a milking stand or put a halter on her and tie her up to a fence post where she can eat a bucket of grain or hay while you milk her. If she's not halter trained, she might follow you a short distance to a bucket of grain.

Clean her udder and teats. You can use baby wipes, followed by dry paper towels. Commercial dairy wipes can be purchased online. Wipe down her udder and teats until the baby wipes remain clean after wiping her teats. Then dry her udder and teats with a clean paper towel.

Milk the first squeeze of milk out onto the ground. Bacteria tends to collect around the teat opening. Milking the first squeeze of milk onto the ground gets rid of this first milk and reduces the chance of bacteria getting into the milk. Reach up and hold the teat at the top, next to the udder bag, and pinch it closed with your thumb and forefinger, closing off the teat. This forces the milk down into the teat and it will look full. Then squeeze from the top down forcing the milk down and out onto the ground. Milk one squeeze out onto the ground from each teat.

Now you are free to collect the milk. Place a clean, dry, stainless steel, seamless bucket under her udder and begin milking away. A cow has four teats. Most people milk two teats at once on one side, alternating squeezes from first one teat then the other. Some squeeze both at the same time. Another way to speed things up is to pair up and milk the cow with one adult and one child. Pair up and each take a side of two teats. Adults usually milk faster and better, but the children need the practice, so halfway switch sides to make sure that each quarter of the udder is milked out completely. Milking in pairs also keeps spirits up and cuts milking time in half!

Filter and cool the milk. When milking is done, one person immediately walks the bucket of milk into the house while the other person puts udder cream on the cow's teats if needed, then walks the cow back to the pasture. Once inside the house, the milk is strained to remove hairs. Two washable coffee filters, double layered, makes a good filter to remove any unwanted hairs from the cow. The milk is poured through the filters directly into storage jars, such as half-gallon Mason jars. Then the milk is immediately chilled down in the fridge.

Then immediately wash and dry all the milking equipment! This is important, too, because you cannot allow dirty milking equipment to sit around. You will also need the equipment fresh, clean and DRY twice a day. Owning only one milking bucket and two coffee strainers forces you to wash them immediately instead of allowing any equipment to sit around dirty. The next day, when the cream rises to the top, carefully ladle the cream off into smaller jars for butter and ice cream.

To better understand the milking process for larger farms that use milking equipment, I highly recommend you watch the DVD "Chore Time" produced by the Farm-to-Consumer Legal Defense Fund. It is a complete guide to raw milk production. On these two DVDs, Tim Wightman (founding board member and Board President) walks the viewer through milk house design, parlor design, milking, heifer training, processing milk, making cream and the clean-up process.

Making Butter and Buttermilk

Making butter and buttermilk is a lot of fun! It also produces a lot of butter. From a gallon and a half of whole milk, you will usually end up with almost ¾ of a pound of butter, or the equivalent of 3 sticks of butter. You will need a food processor to whip the butter to the right consistency where the cream begins to churn and collect into clumps of butter. Set the jars of whole milk in the fridge overnight so the cream will rise to the top. Try not to shake or jostle the jars as you remove them from the fridge the next day. Using a small ladle, carefully skim the cream off the top and into a jar. Three half gallon jars of whole milk should yield about a quart of cream. This cream may be thick in some spots. That's fine.

Pour the quart of cream into the food processor. Add 1 tsp of finely ground sea salt if desired. Blend on low speed for 10 minutes. While the butter is churning, prepare a medium sized bowl half full of ice water and ice cubes.

Stop the food processor and open to check for clumps of butter. If the cream looks like whipped cream, it's not ready yet. Butter that is ready will have turned darker yellow and will have separated from the liquid in the cream. It will look like there are clumps of half-melted butter floating on top of skim milk. If you gather some of this lumpy butter on a spoon, it will also lump together and pile up thick on the spoon. If the butter is not ready, run the food processor on high speed for a few minutes more.

When the butter is ready, pour this lumpy butter and watery liquid through a reusable coffee filter into a separate bowl to catch the buttermilk (NOT the bowl of ice water). This watery liquid is thin buttermilk. Save for later. It is excellent for making cornbread and pancakes.

Remove ice cubes from the bowl of ice water! Then dump the lumpy butter from the strainer into the bowl of cold water. Allow the butter to sit in the cold water for a minute or two, or place in the fridge for only a few minutes. This will firm up the butter, but you do not want it to completely harden. Pour off the cold water and press the butter with a spatula. Keep pressing the butter until most of the water has been removed (there is no need to save this water).

It is not necessary to remove all the water from the butter, but remove as much as you can. At this stage, the more you mess with the butter, the messier it gets. Then scoop this butter into a container and place in the fridge. Done!

Whey and Yogurt Cheese

Yogurt can be strained to create a soft, creamy, and tart "cream cheese." The liquid that is strained from this yogurt is called whey and can be used to boost lacto-fermented vegetables. Either make or purchase a one-quart container of plain whole milk yogurt. Using a clean dishtowel or butter muslin, scoop plain yogurt into the cloth and tie up all four corners around the handle of a long wooden spoon. Hang the bundle inside an empty plastic water pitcher, laying the wooden spoon handle across the top of the pitcher to hold the bundle of yogurt off of the bottom. The bundle of yogurt should be hanging several inches above the bottom of the pitcher. Place pitcher in the fridge overnight to drain. It will catch the liquid whey as it slowly drains from the bag. In the morning, untie the bundle and scoop the contents into a clean container with a lid. Store in the fridge. Pour the whey into a jar and store in the refrigerator. This yogurt cheese can be flavored with garlic, onion, or with dill to make a creamy spread or dip.

Making basic cheese

This is a simple recipe for homemade cheese. The possibilities for home cheese-making are endless. I highly recommend the resource "Home Cheese Making" by Ricki Carroll. Her website, The New England Cheesemaking Supply Company has loads of resources, equipment, and cultures for home cheese making.

Begin with two gallons of whole, fresh cow's milk in a deep large pot. (This recipe will not work with ultra-heat treated, pasteurized, milk). Gently warm the milk on low heat, approximately 100 degrees Fahrenheit, while stirring gently. Add ½ teaspoon of liquid rennet and stir gently into the milk.

After stirring for one minute, turn off heat, return the lid to the pot and let sit for 45 minutes. This is the stage where the milk will begin to separate from the whey.

When the milk has separated, it will look like you have white gelatin sitting in a pot of clear liquid whey. With a long butter knife, make long vertical slices into the white gelatin one inch apart. Turn the pot 90 degrees and make another set of slices perpendicular to the first set. Line a mixing bowl with a single layer of cheese cloth. Using a cheese strainer (or ladle) scoop up the curds into the mixing bowl, leaving the liquid in the pot. Generously sprinkle the cheese curds with 1-2 tablespoons of fine sea salt and stir. Tie up the four corners of the cheese cloth to an upper kitchen cabinet handle, leaving the bowl beneath to catch the remaining whey. Let drip for several hours or longer.

When the bundle stops dripping, pour off the whey into a jar for later use if desired. Untie the cheese cloth and place the curds into a mixing bowl. Use your hands or a spatula to break up the curds. Add more salt if desired. These curds are ready to eat. Homemade cottage cheese can be made by crumbling the curds into a mixing bowl and covering generously with cream.

To make a firm block of cheese, take the same curds, return them to the cheese cloth and press them in a cheese press using about 10 pounds of pressure. Let the cheese stay under pressure for an hour or more. If you do not have a cheese press, sandwich the curds in the cloth between two cutting boards, with a weight on top. Place this make-shift cheese press on a baking sheet to catch additional whey.

Homemade Ice Cream

You will need an ice cream maker but homemade ice cream is well worth it. White sugar will produce ice cream that tastes like store-bought ice cream. Using brown sugar or turbinado sugar will produce an ice cream that tastes like butter-pecan. To make a simple vanilla ice cream, combine the following ingredients in a half gallon jar then place in the fridge prior to placing in the ice cream maker. The mixture needs to be as cold as possible, and still be a liquid, before placing in the ice cream maker.

Commercial ice cream contains many types of gums and thickeners. To make homemade ice cream as creamy as store-bought, I use a little trick that incorporates unflavored gelatin into the ice cream. This has the added benefit of working grass-fed bovine gelatin into our diet, which is good for joints and tendons. I also add egg yolks from our chickens or from a farmer's market. It is important that they are not eggs from chickens raised in commercial farms.

Start by dissolving one tablespoon of granulated bovine gelatin in two to four tablespoons of hot water. Let this mixture cool before adding three farm fresh egg yolks. Add one cup of brown or turbinado sugar, two tablespoons vanilla extract, and stir thoroughly. If you have vanilla beans on hand, the seeds from one bean will add additional flavor and character to the appearance. Add four cups heavy cream or fresh raw milk cream. Place the mixture back in the fridge to cool. Set up your ice cream machine and follow manufacturer's instructions.

Vanilla Ice Cream

1 tbsp. gelatin dissolved in 2-4 tbsp. hot water
3 egg yolks
2 tbsp. vanilla extract
1 cup sugar
*Seeds from 1 vanilla bean (optional)
4 cups heavy cream (1 quart)

Chocolate Ice Cream: Follow recipe above but add only 1 tbsp. vanilla, and add 2 tbsp. cocoa powder

Blueberry Ice Cream: only 1 tbsp. vanilla, and add 1 cup fresh or frozen blueberries

Eggs

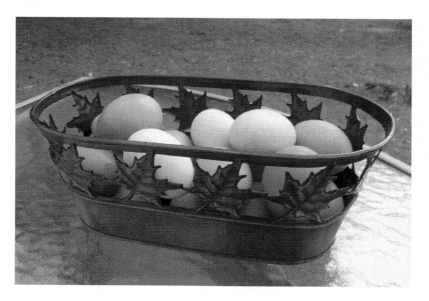

It's unfair what Western culture has done to eggs. Eggs are such a rich and versatile food! Eggs are affordable and an essential food for families. Eggs are a complete food, and the yolk requires almost no digestion. Raw yolks from healthy hens are a perfect first food for babies. Dr. Natasha Campbell-McBride writes that "Eggs are one of the most nourishing and easy-to-digest foods on the planet. Raw egg yolk has been compared with human breast milk because it can be absorbed almost 100% without needing digestion."[28] Eggs are also rich in vitamins B1, B2, B6, B12, A, D and Biotin, most essential fatty acids, zinc and magnesium.[29]

Buy eggs from a farm that you trust. I recommend that all families purchasing meat, eggs, or milk visit the farm that is raising their food and see the animals. Learn to recognize healthy animals. Chickens like to wander around in grass or shrubs and hunt for insects. Ducks need a small pond to bathe and swim in to stay clean. Chickens raised in the sun and fresh air have better immune systems that help them stay healthy. The possibility of these hens having salmonella is far lower than battery-produced eggs from hens kept in cages. Chickens get sick with salmonella from eating grain that has been contaminated with feces from rats that carry salmonella. If you haven't seen the farm or place where the chickens are raised, don't eat the eggs raw. Cook them thoroughly.

If your family doesn't like scrambled eggs for breakfast, try an old tradition: custard. It is an absolute crying shame that eggs, butter and cream were disregarded because they used to be the foundation for every rich and creamy dessert. To me, dessert devoid of cream and eggs is useless. You need the rich fats and protein in eggs and cream to balance the sugar. Nobody wants to eat sugar by itself. Let us indulge for a moment. In my house, nobody likes the idea of custard because everyone for the last fifty years has made it wrong – low fat and watery. Why bother? So, I took an old tradition and made it new: cream, eggs, vanilla and sugar. I mixed together a lot of vanilla, heavy whipping cream, about a half-dozen eggs, and some sugar. I call it Vanilla Pie, and everybody loves it! On another occasion, I mashed six very ripe bananas, four eggs, some sugar and cream and made a delicious banana pudding. Eggs are amazing. I love them. I also combine eggs, milk, cream, spices, and bake that into a delicious pumpkin pie. The recipes for these follow this section. Love your eggs. They will love you back.

The Cholesterol Myth

Eggs are rich in cholesterol. We don't know enough about cholesterol to be condemning every food that contains cholesterol. If God put cholesterol naturally in our food, I say we leave it there and enjoy it. I also find it interesting that God designed humans to have an egg sac full of cholesterol sitting right next to the developing embryo at its most vulnerable stage of development. That's not an accident. It's time we admit that dietary cholesterol and blood cholesterol are not the same thing. Dr. Campbell-McBride writes that, "The majority of people do not know that 85% of blood cholesterol does not come from food but is produced by the liver in response to consumption of processed carbohydrates and sugar. So, these are the foods to avoid to protect your heart, not the eggs."[30]

Ron Schimd, ND, tells us in *The Untold Story of Milk*, "Today, most researchers admit that dietary cholesterol has only a slight influence on cholesterol levels in the blood – despite broad public acceptance of the dictum that we should restrict intake of cholesterol – because the body's cholesterol level is regulated in the liver according to individual needs. The more cholesterol we eat, the less the liver makes, and vice-versa. Even an extreme diet generally lowers cholesterol by no more than about ten percent in the short run. I've observed that extended periods of protein deficiency in people who follow vegetarian or near vegetarian diets can lower cholesterol perhaps a bit more, even down to levels around 150 mg/dl for some people. This may be due to the lack of protein, needed for the production of cholesterol. (These patients are then distressed to learn that low cholesterol levels are a strong risk factor for cancer.)"[31]

I find the story of how cholesterol became demonized quite interesting, actually. I believe we made a heroic but enormous goof. Looking at the numbers, we saw people dying of heart attacks and, at the same time, saw numbers that these people had elevated levels of blood cholesterol. Rightly concerned, we made the wrong connection that blood cholesterol must be bad for us. It's sort of like arriving to the scene of an accident and watching the ambulance and first responders whisk away all the injured people to the hospital. A child, not knowing who the first responders are or where they're taking the injured, would be dreadfully concerned about the people *taking away* the injured. "Who are they? Why are they taking away the people that need help? Somebody stop them!" In a fashion, we made the same mistake. Every auto accident will have an ambulance and first responders. That doesn't mean they caused the accident. Raised blood cholesterol levels are an indicator, not a cause. But remember, God designed them to be given to embryos in their most vulnerable state. The liver naturally produces blood cholesterol. What if blood cholesterol is our body's first-responders, the first on scene to an area of our body that needs help? Wouldn't we be foolish to try to remove them?

Misconceptions about cholesterol keep people from enjoying eggs. "Many of you believe that cholesterol in foods can cause heart disease and wonder how unprocessed milk, butter and cream can be good for us since they are rich in animal fats and cholesterol. My answer is simple: 'Because animal fats and cholesterol are good for you.'" -Ron Schmid, ND.

Egg Drop Soup

Heat 1 cup of roast chicken drippings on the stove in a pot. Add 4 cups of water and bring to a boil. Taste and add more drippings if too watery or add water if it's too salty. In a separate small cup, add one teaspoon cornstarch and two teaspoons of water; mix until a thin paste forms. Add two more tablespoons of water to the paste, stir thoroughly, and then add to the pot of broth, stirring as you add. Continue to boil until the broth thickens. A spoon dipped in the broth will coat the spoon when done properly. Once the broth has thickened, remove from heat. Break two eggs into a cereal bowl and scramble. Add raw scrambled eggs to the broth while stirring slowly. Place back on medium heat until eggs are fully cooked, about 1-2 minutes.

Simple Eggnog

1 ½ cups cream
4 egg yolks from healthy, free range chickens
½ tsp. vanilla extract
Nutmeg 1/8 tsp.
Sugar ¾ cup

Mix ingredients with stick blender and strain to remove large particles of undissolved spices and sugar. Add ¼ cup of milk to thin to desired consistency.

Vanilla Pie

The first time I made this at home, I told my family I made a custard for dessert. Nobody ate it. They wouldn't even taste it! The second time I made it, I got a little smarter. I made the same exact recipe but I told everyone I made Vanilla Pie for dessert. It disappeared within a day. Everybody loved it! So this recipe is called Vanilla Pie, even though it is really a custard... a delicious one!

For the crust:
½ cup softened pork lard or 1 stick softened butter
2 cups flour
¼ tsp. salt

Preheat oven to 350F. In a mixing bowl, mix softened butter or lard, flour, and salt with a fork until a soft dough forms. It should hold together when pressed in your hand, but not be too greasy. If too greasy, add a little more flour. If too dry and doesn't hold together, add a little more softened butter or lard. Do not add water to the dough, as this makes dumplings and not crunchy pie crust. To make a firm dough, place in the fridge for a few minutes to chill the dough.

Roll dough with a rolling pin to create a circle about 2" wider than the pie dish on all sides. Press dough into a glass baking dish. Press as evenly as possible, using the dough to cover the entire inside of the dish. Trim the top of the crust so it is even with the top of the pie dish, or fold over into a decorative edge along the rim of the pie dish.

For the custard:
1 cup sugar
3 tbsp. flour
4-5 eggs
1 ½ tbsp. vanilla extract
¾ cup softened butter
1 cup heavy whipping cream

In a mixing bowl, combine the sugar and flour. Stir thoroughly. Add eggs and vanilla extract, and stir again. Add softened butter and mix thoroughly with a stick blender. Fold in heavy whipping cream and mix again with stick blender until smooth. Pour into uncooked pie crust and bake for 45-50 minutes or until toothpick inserted in center comes out clean.

Banana Pie

For the crust:
1 stick softened butter or pork lard
2 cups flour
¼ tsp. salt

Preheat oven to 350F. In a mixing bowl, mix softened butter or lard, flour, and salt with a fork until a soft dough forms. It should hold together when pressed in your hand, but not be too greasy. If too greasy, add a little more flour. If too dry and doesn't hold together, add a little more softened butter or lard. Do not add water to the dough, as this makes dumplings and not crunchy pie crust. To make a firm dough, place in the fridge for a few minutes to chill the dough.

Roll dough with a rolling pin to create a circle about 2" wider than the pie dish on all sides. Press dough into a glass baking dish. Press as evenly as possible, using the dough to cover the entire inside of the dish. Trim the top of the crust so it is even with the top of the pie dish, or fold over into a decorative edge along the rim of the pie dish.

For the filling:
1 stick (1/2 cup) of softened butter or coconut oil
6 ripe bananas (they should have a few black speckles on the peel)
1 cup sugar
4 eggs
1 cup cream

Preheat oven to 350F. Spray a glass pie dish with oil or rub with butter. On the stove, in a medium pot, melt the butter on medium-low heat. Add bananas and mash with a potato masher. Add sugar and stir until dissolved. Remove from heat. Wait for mixture to cool a few minutes, about 5 minutes. Stir in the eggs and cream. Mix with stick blender until smooth. Pour into uncooked pie crust and bake at 350F for 45-50 minutes or until toothpick inserted in center comes out clean.

Real Pumpkin Pie

For the crust:
1 stick softened butter or pork lard
2 cups flour
¼ tsp. salt
*Optional maple syrup, about ¼ cup

For the filling:
3 cups cooked pumpkin (See recipe: How to preserve pumpkin)
3/4 cup sugar
1 tsp. cinnamon
½ tsp. ground ginger
¼ tsp. ground cloves
¼ tsp. ground nutmeg
3 eggs
1 cup heavy cream

Preheat oven to 350F. In a mixing bowl, mix softened butter or lard, flour, and salt with a fork until a soft dough forms. It should hold together when pressed in your hand, but not be too greasy. If too greasy, add a little more flour. If too dry and doesn't hold together, add a little more softened butter or lard. Do not add water to the dough, as this makes dumplings and not crunchy pie crust. To make a firm dough, place in the fridge for a few minutes to chill the dough.

Roll dough with a rolling pin to create a circle about 2" wider than the pie dish on all sides. Press dough into a glass baking dish. Press as evenly as possible, using the dough to cover the entire inside of the dish. Trim the top of the crust so it is even with the top of the pie dish, or fold over into a decorative edge along the rim of the pie dish. Optional: drizzle the crust with maple syrup.

In a large mixing bowl, stir sugar into cooked pumpkin. Add spices by sprinkling on top of pumpkin mixture and stir thoroughly (*2 tsp. of the Pumpkin Pie Spice recipe in the herbs section will replace the spices). Add eggs and cream and stir again. If mixture is lumpy, blend with stick blender until smooth.

Pour on top of unbaked crust and bake at 350F for 45-50 minutes or until toothpick inserted in center comes out clean.

PLANT FOODS

Fruit (of the plant)

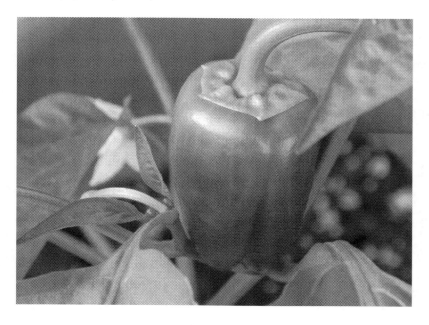

Fruits of the plant have been one of mankind's favorite foods, all the way back to Genesis. There are so many to choose from: pumpkin, peppers, apples, tomatoes... They are bursting with flavor and often can carry an entire dish. Examples include apple pie and tomato sauce. Fruits can be expensive to purchase at the grocery store so it's important to know where to buy affordable fruit. U-pick farms are an excellent source of fresh fruit that can be at reasonable prices. Visiting farmer's markets and buying bulk can help keep the costs down. Especially if you're going to cook or render the fruit in a short period of time. Growing your own fruit trees can yield gallons of fresh fruit but be prepared for excess and how to store them when the crops come into season.

Dried vegetables (dehydrated or freeze dried) retain much more of their nutrients than canned or frozen. Since shipping fees are determined by weight, it doesn't make sense to ship metal cans and vegetables packed in water across the country, adding to the cost. Dehydrated vegetables are lighter and more nutritious. They are also an affordable option purchased in bulk.

How to preserve pumpkin & winter squash

Many people do not realize that all pumpkins are edible and can be cooked down and frozen for later use. Some pumpkins are small with darker, sweeter flesh perfect for making pumpkin pies. Others are large and have light yellow flesh that taste similar to yellow crookneck squash or zucchini once it has been cooked. These are great for use in soups, stews and muffins. Many pumpkin patches will often give away leftover pumpkins when they close for the fall. These lumpy, misshapen, "ugly" pumpkins are perfect for cooking down and storing for later use. Make sure you select a pumpkin that is firm with no soft spots. Soft spots on the outside of the pumpkin usually mean mold on the inside.

There are two ways to cook pumpkin. The first method is to roast the pumpkin in the oven, then scoop out the soft, cooked flesh. The other method is cutting the pumpkin into large chunks and boiling in hot water until soft and tender. Other types of hard winter squash can be roasted this way as well, such as acorn squash or butternut squash.

Roasting in the oven is my personal favorite. Roasting breaks down the natural sugars in the pumpkin lending a sweeter, fuller flavor. Plus, pumpkin is so much easier to slice once it's cooked! Preheat the oven to 350° while prepping the pumpkin for roasting. (Prepping the pumpkin is optional but helps reduce cleanup time. To roast a pumpkin whole without cutting it at all, prick the peeling a few times with a fork to let steam escape.) To prep the pumpkin for roasting, cut a hole in the top and remove the stem and the seeds. This has the advantage of letting you see the condition of the flesh inside. Make sure the flesh is still fresh and moist, not dried up or moldy. If so, throw it away or feed it to chickens.

Place on a baking sheet and bake at 350° for 45 to 60 minutes. Larger pumpkins (10 pounds or more) may require an hour and a half or more to roast. Baking time depends on the thickness of the pumpkin walls; thicker walls mean more roasting time required. To reduce roasting time, slice the entire pumpkin in half and place cut side down on a baking sheet.

Boiling pumpkin in hot water is quicker but does take more time to slice the pumpkin into chunks first. After cutting a hole in the top and removing the stem and seeds, slice the pumpkin lengthwise into long strips about 1 to 2 inches thick. Strips longer than 8 inches can be cut in half. Boil the chunks of pumpkin in a large pot of hot water for 20 to 25 minutes, or until soft and tender.

Once the pieces of pumpkin have been cooked, set them aside for a few minutes to cool. Take a large metal spoon and scrape the flesh away from the peeling. This should be easy now that the pumpkin is cooked. The cooked pumpkin can be scooped into containers or plastic bags and frozen for later use. To obtain a finer texture, process in a food processor or with a stick blender until smooth. The leftover peeling and seeds can be given to chickens as a tasty snack.

Tomato Sauce

8 medium ripe tomatoes
2 tsp. minced garlic, or 2-3 cloves fresh minced garlic
2 tsp. sea salt
2 tsp. dried oregano
2 tsp. dried basil

Bring a small pot of water about 4 inches deep to a boil and cut an "X" in bottom of tomatoes. Cut out stem sections. Soak tomatoes in boiling water for 30-45 seconds. Allow to cool and begin peeling at the X. Peel should slip off easily.

Cut whole tomatoes in half or in quarters. Place peeled tomatoes in empty pot. Gently smash with potato masher. Bring to boil. Add garlic, salt and spices. Simmer until tomatoes are soft. Sauce is done!

Maple & Butter Acorn Squash

Cut a large squash in half and scoop out the seeds. Place both halves, cut side up, in a baking dish. Add two tablespoons of butter and 1/3 cup of maple syrup to the center of the cut halves. Bake at 350F for 45 minutes or until fork tender. Another great flavor combination for acorn squash filling is cranberries and honey.

Vanilla Extract

Begin with one 750ml high-quality bottle of potato vodka and add 6 whole vanilla beans that have been scored and sliced down the long axis of the bean. Do not remove the seeds. Allow them to steep in the vodka for a minimum 3 weeks before using. Store indefinitely.

Strawberries and Cream, or Peaches and Cream

Start with one quart of fresh ripe strawberries. Destem the strawberries and slice into quarters. Pour one cup of cream over the strawberries. Very ripe strawberries should not need any sugar but 1-2 tablespoons can be added if necessary.

For peaches and cream, prepare the peaches by slicing in half and removing the pit. Slice the halved peaches to ½ to ¾ inch slices. Pour cream over the peaches. Add sugar to taste. For spiced peaches and cream, sprinkle the peaches and cream lightly with cinnamon and nutmeg.

Stalks and Leaves

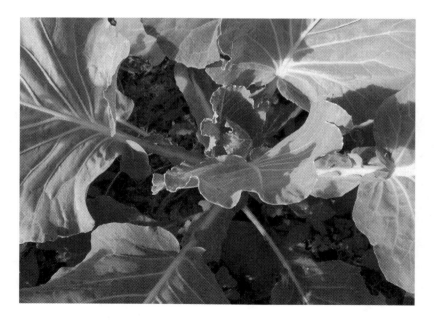

Vegetable stalks and leaves, such as collards, broccoli stems, and kale need a lot of flavor added to them. They are typically bland in flavor or may even have a sharp bite, such as collard or turnip greens. The only exception to this list is celery, which is highly aromatic and flavorful, so much so that it is actually sold as a spice and is one of the big three ingredients in bone broths. However, broccoli stems, brussels stems, and most everything else in the *brassica* family needs some fat and flavor. These stalks need meat drippings, healthy animal fats, and herbs. I wouldn't serve these items as a dish by themselves, but they pair wonderfully with other tender vegetables, with hot sauce, in stuffing and casseroles, and in creamy dips like the ones listed below.

Chopping and using celery, collards, turnip greens

Collards and turnip greens from a fruit stand can be massive! When chopping and slicing large leafy greens, roll the pile of leaves into a roll about 2-3 inches thick, and make small slices about half an inch wide starting at the tip and working toward the root.

Creamy Greens Dip, Spinach, Kale, Collards

To get my children to eat more dark, leafy greens, I made a creamy dip to serve with corn chips. Start with a creamy cheese base such as farm fresh ricotta cheese or one package (8 oz.) of cream cheese. Melt the cheese in a frying pan with one or two tablespoons of butter. Add 1/2 cup of diced leafy greens of your choice such as fresh spinach, kale, collard greens, or turnip greens. Heat on medium heat and stir until the greens become tender and melt into the cheese and butter. Sprinkle with salt, onion powder, and garlic to taste. Parmesan cheese or seasoned salt are other options for seasoning.

Veggies cooked in drippings

I'm convinced people don't like vegetables because they are not cooked in enough flavor. Some of our favorite ways of cooking vegetables are with several tablespoons of roast chicken drippings, roast beef drippings, or turkey drippings. Sautee vegetables in a frying pan with the drippings until tender, making sure you include 1-2 tablespoons of the fat layer at the top of the drippings jar.

Alfredo Sauce and Veggies

Another great way to eat vegetables is to serve them smothered in creamy alfredo sauce. To make a simple alfredo sauce, melt two tablespoons of butter in a frying pan. Add ½ - ¾ cup of heavy whipping cream, ½ cup of parmesan cheese, 1 tsp. lemon juice, and sprinkle with salt and pepper to taste. Stir until ingredients are thoroughly mixed and pour onto steamed vegetables.

Roots and Tubers

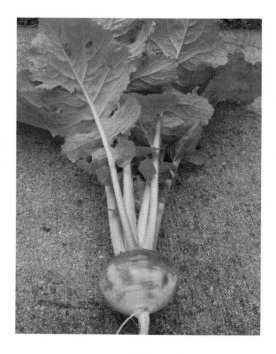

Roots and tubers are the cornerstone of flavor when it comes to vegetables. Most roots are so heavily flavored that people do not eat them by themselves, such as onions, garlic, beets, radishes, and turnips. One of the best ways to draw out their flavor and release the natural sugars is to roast them in the oven. Roots that naturally contain a lot of sugar, such as carrots, onions and garlic can be slow roasted to caramelize the natural sugars. Caramelizing onions and garlic breaks down the sugar and tones down the potency. Toss the vegetables in a few tablespoons of oil before roasting. *The Roasted Vegetable,* by Andrea Chesman, is a great resource on how to coax flavors out of roasted vegetables.

Caramelized Onions

Remove the outer husk of one large onion and cut into thin slices. Pan fry in 2-3 tablespoons of butter on medium-low heat until the onions become translucent and begin to brown. Stir thoroughly to coat each piece with oil. As the onions begin to brown, you will notice a distinct change in the aroma from a raw onion smell to a rich savory sweet tone. When the onions are soft and browned, remove from heat. These are perfect added to hamburgers, sour cream or beef broth.

Oven Roasted Garlic

Take four whole heads of garlic and slice about half an inch of the top to reveal the tops of the cloves. Place the clusters cut side up in a roasting dish. Drizzle liberally with olive oil. Bake at 350F for 30-40 minutes or until garlic cloves are soft. Remove from oven and allow to cool for 15 minutes. Once cool, the cloves will easily slip out of the heads of garlic. Place the cloves and remaining olive oil from the baking pan in a jar and store in the fridge. Use in recipes that call for garlic, such as salads and dips. This garlic will have a sweeter flavor and less bite.

Legumes and Grains

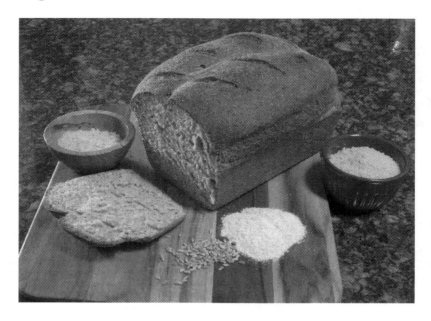

"the finest kernels of wheat..." Deuteronomy 32:14

Did you know that more than 30 nutrients are lost in the commercial milling process of wheat? It seems like an unnecessary step to home-grind flour, with so many types of flour available at the supermarket. However, commercially milled flour is not the same as home-ground flour – not even close. Communities used to mill their flour in local stone mills. Only the wealthy had the opportunity to buy white, refined flour because it was a labor-intensive process to remove the bran and germ from the flour. In 1878, a new invention changed the history of flour forever. The new steel roller sifted the bran and germ out of whole ground wheat and the result was a finely ground white flour that was quickly embraced by communities everywhere.[32] It took almost forty years before researchers connected the rise in diseases to the loss of B vitamins and iron from the missing bran and germ. In 1941, the government stepped in and mandated the "enrichment" of commercially milled flour, but only a fraction of the lost nutrients is replaced in enriched flour.

The importance of whole-grain wheat is vital to understand for proper nutrition. Sue Becker explains about the benefits of fresh-milled wheat in her book, *The Essential Home-Ground Flour Book*. In a wheat kernel, the chaff is the outer husk of the seed. It is inedible and is threshed and winnowed to remove the chaff from the seed. The rest of the seed is called the "wheat berry." The bran is the next outer layer of the wheat berry and coats and protects the seed from spoilage. The germ is the spot where the seed germinates and sprouts. In refined flour, the bran and germ are discarded. This is unfortunate because the bran and germ contain many B vitamins and enzymes contained within the wheat kernel. The germ is the most nutrient-dense part of the seed and contains essential fatty acids, vitamin E, the bulk of the B vitamins, antioxidants, and minerals.[33] Because fresh milled flour contains all the bran, eating bread made from fresh-ground flour does not lead to constipation. By grinding the whole wheat berry, the flour includes all the bran, and so all the fiber.

To this day, our youngest daughter has asthmatic symptoms and an "allergy" to commercially processed wheat, even though she does not have an actual wheat allergy. We went gluten-free for several years before trying home-ground flour. We saw the largest improvement in her health when we bought a home grain mill. We learned that we can make an endless variety of breads, kneaded dough and sandwich loaves, rolls, cookies, cakes, crackers and more out of home-ground flour... and she does not have any negative reaction. As it turns out, it wasn't the gluten that was bothering her. Commercially-milled flour has several additives to bleach and oxidize the flour, such as benzoyl peroxide as a bleaching agent; calcium carbonate, calcium sulfate, or dicalcium phosphate to neutralize the benzoyl peroxide, and potassium bromate to oxidize and strengthen the gluten structure.[34] We are happy to report that our daughter can eat anything we make at home with fresh-milled flour with no reaction at all.

The price of a mill can be intimidating for some families. We spent about $220 for our mill, a Wondermill. Good news – the whole wheat berries are not expensive at all! We purchase our wheat berries in bulk, at about $1.50 per pound. And that's for organic wheat berries. Using about 20 pounds of wheat per month for home baking, that cost comes to about $30 per month for all of our wheat and bread products. That price does not include yeast or sugar, but I still think we come out ahead. Especially considering how much healthier we are, and that we do not buy gluten-free products any more. Milling fresh wheat berries is also a time saver because you do not have to sift the flour. It comes out of the mill nice and fluffy.

There are several types of wheat berries that can be purchased. As a general rule of thumb, hard wheat berries are better at developing gluten for breads that require kneading, such as sandwich bread, rolls and baguettes. Soft wheat berries are better for breads and cakes that will not be kneaded, such as muffins and cookies.

Leavening Agents

It's important to understand how different leavening agents work. Bakers use different leavening (rising) agents. Yeast and baking powder (also baking soda) are used to make bread rise. As a general rule of thumb, yeast allows bread to rise *outside* the oven. Baking powder is activated *inside* the oven. When working with yeast, give the dough enough time to rise to its finished shape before baking. In other words, once you place it in the oven, it's not going to rise any more. Don't mix a dough together containing only yeast as a leavening agent, then place it half-risen in the oven expecting it to continue to rise. It won't. Baking powder is activated by the heat and steam from the bread, causing the bread to rise in the oven.

Fermenting Bread

Eggs enrich bread, adding valuable fats and flavor to the bread. This is useful for cakes, muffins and cookies, but for crisp, crunchy loaves of bread, such as French bread, you will need ample time to allow the yeast to work. Professionals will make a *pate fermentee* or starter for the dough and refrigerate it overnight. This starter is mixed with the rest of the flour in the morning, lending rich flavor to the final loaf of bread. For more detailed information about properly forming dough and kneaded breads, such as French bread, focaccia, and baguettes, see *The Bread Baker's Apprentice* by Peter Reinhart.

Basic Sandwich Bread and Rolls

I use the same recipe for sandwich bread and rolls, adding a little extra sugar for rolls. This bread is enriched with eggs.

½ cup warm water
2 ½ tsp. quick-rising yeast
1 tbsp. oil
1 tbsp. sugar or honey
2 eggs
1 tsp. salt
3-3 ½ cups fresh-milled flour, hard wheat

In a mixing bowl, add water and yeast. Stir thoroughly until yeast dissolves. Add oil, honey, eggs and salt. Mix thoroughly. Add flour one cup at a time and mix until soft dough forms. I've found that mixing is easier using a wooden spatula or stiff wooden spoon. Allow to rest for 15 minutes at room temperature.

To knead dough: Have about ½-1 cup extra flour available. Lightly sprinkle a clean countertop with flour. Move dough to countertop and begin folding the dough in half and then press down. Fold the dough in half towards you and press down with both hands. Turn the dough 90 degrees, then fold in half and press down again. Repeat this process until the dough is thoroughly mixed. Sprinkle dough with more flour if it becomes sticky. If dough is dry and crumbly, add water one tablespoon at a time and knead thoroughly. Repeat this process for 5 minutes or until dough becomes smooth and elastic. It will be elastic when pressed with a thumb and the dough springs back.

Using the wooden spatula, scrape up the dough and return to mixing bowl. Cover with plastic wrap or cloth and let rise for 1 hour or until doubled in size.

Butter or oil a loaf pan. Gently shape dough to a long, thick log as long as the loaf pan. Move dough to the loaf pan and let rise until the top of dough rises above the pan by about ½ inch. Bake at 350 for 30 minutes or until top has lightly browned. Remove from bread pan and cool on a wire rack.

Sweet Rolls

Follow the recipe for Basic Sandwich Bread but add an extra tbsp. of sugar or honey. For holiday breads, or stuffed breads, spices can also be added in this step, such as a sprinkle of cinnamon or cloves. To shape into rolls, roll dough into a log about 2-3 inches thick. Divide dough into equal sections about 2 inches in diameter. Butter or oil a muffin tray. Place one ball of dough in each muffin cup. Let rise in muffin tray until tops rise above the tray. Bake at 350 for 25-30 minutes.

Quick Flatbread Crust

4 cups fresh-milled flour, hard or soft wheat
1 tsp. salt
1/2 tsp. baking soda
4 tbsp. olive oil
½ to 1 cup water

Combine flour, salt and baking soda in bowl and mix thoroughly. Add olive oil and ¾ cup of water and mix with stiff wooden spoon. Knead until the flour creates a stiff dough, adding additional water if necessary. Cut dough in half. Roll each half out onto hard surface until ¼ inch thick. Bake about 15 min at 400 degrees. Top with sauce, cheese and vegetables of your choice. Bake for an additional 10 minutes until vegetables and cheese have browned. Makes 2 flatbreads.

Homemade Stuffing

1 loaf of sandwich bread
Drippings from roast chicken or turkey
1 ½ cups chopped celery
2 thinly sliced carrots
1 diced small onion, or 2 tbsp. dry minced onion
Salt and butter to taste

Cut one loaf of sandwich bread into 1 inch cubes. Save drippings from chicken or turkey, about ½ to 1 cup. Boil chopped celery, carrots and onion in water until soft. Drain water from celery and vegetables, setting aside a few cups of this water to add to chicken or turkey drippings. In a separate bowl, add just enough celery water to chicken or turkey drippings to create about 1 cup of hot broth. Add cooked celery and vegetables to bread cubes. Pour broth over bread cubes and vegetables, just enough to moisten the bread cubes and stir thoroughly. Add salt and butter to taste.

Soaking & cooking Beans

Green beans, butter beans, dried beans... there are a lot to choose from! Green beans are the young, tender pods that are picked green before the seeds inside have a chance to grow large and mature. Butter beans are the soft, young seeds that are picked green, but have had the time to swell in the pod and form large beans. A familiar type of butter bean is the frozen lima bean available in the grocery store. These butter beans are soft, fresh and only require a quick cooking time in some butter or oil, hence the name "butter beans." Dried beans are harvested after the entire bean pod and seeds inside have grown to full maturity, then allowed to dry and the pods turned brown. These hard, dried beans can be a variety of colors from black, brown, speckled, white, golden, and red. They are beautiful and store for a year or so at room temperature.

Dried beans are affordable and loaded with fiber and nutrients. To use dried beans, they must be soaked in water overnight. First, sort the beans by allowing 2 cups of beans to fall slowly over your hand into a bowl. Look over the beans carefully for unusable beans or small rocks. Place dried beans in a large mixing bowl. Fill the bowl with water, submersing the beans with an extra two inches of water above the beans. They will double in size overnight. The next day, pour off the water and rinse the beans. To cook the them, place them in a large pot with enough water to cover the beans. Bring water to a boil, reduce heat, and simmer for at least 4 hours or until tender.

Herbs and Spices

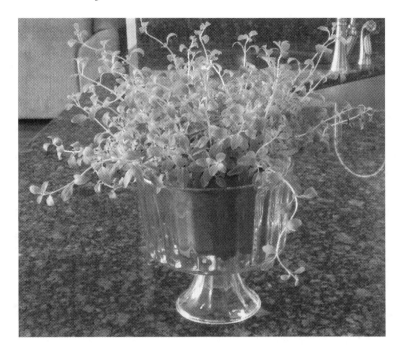

I've found over the years that it's easy to replace pre-mixed ingredients, such as taco seasoning, once you know the primary herb in the flavoring mix. We've done this with many types of dry powders and dressings, such as ranch dressing mix. It can be difficult to find a ranch dressing mix that does not contain MSG, or a dressing that does not contain soybean oil. Here are a few shortcuts we use in the kitchen to replace the seasonings that contain soy or MSG. Also, check the section in "Bone Broths" for spices to replace cream of chicken and cream of mushroom soup.

Ranch Dressing

The main flavor combination in this dressing is dill weed and sour cream. Onion and garlic compliment the flavors and help round out the dressing. The dry ingredients can be premixed and sprinkled onto other foods for a ranch dressing flavor.

1 cup sour cream (or plain milk kefir), ½ tsp. dill weed, ¼ tsp. onion, ¼ tsp. garlic, 1/8 tsp. salt. Add milk to reach desired consistency. For a creamier dressing, add olive oil to desired consistency instead of milk.

Taco Seasoning

You can use many different combinations of spices for taco seasoning as long as you have included cumin. Open the bottle of ground cumin and smell the spice. It smells like tacos! Paprika, chili powder, and onion help round out the flavors. Add more cumin, chili powder and cayenne to add heat to the tacos.

1 tbsp. paprika
2 tsp. powdered onion
1 tsp. powdered garlic
½ tsp. ground cumin
1 tsp. chili powder
1 tsp. sea salt

Pumpkin Pie Spice

4 tsp. cinnamon
2 tsp. ground ginger
1 tsp. ground cloves
1 tsp. ground nutmeg
*(2 tsp. of this mix will replace the spices in the Pumpkin Pie recipe).

Seasoned salt

2 tbsp. sea salt (not course ground)
2 tbsp. powdered onion
1 tsp. smoked paprika

1 tbsp. powdered garlic
1 tsp. dried celery or celery seed

Onion Soup Mix

1/3 cup dried minced onion, or one large fresh onion chopped
1 tsp. sea salt
½ cup beef drippings

LIVING FOODS AND DRINKS

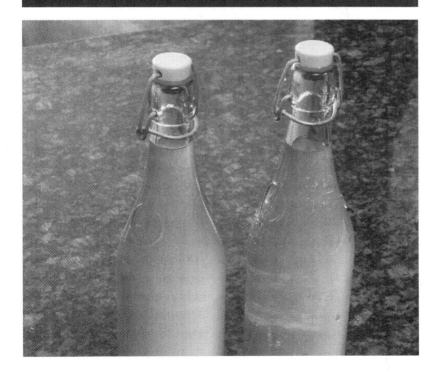

There are many types of living foods that naturally contain beneficial microflora and can be used to strengthen the immune system and heal the gut. There are simply too many to list here. Raw milk dairy products are an obvious choice. They contain the widest variety of beneficial microflora and can be cultured into yogurt, butter, buttermilk, milk kefir, cheeses and ice cream.

Other living foods are created using vegetables or fruit juice. As with all fermented foods, the living foods described in this section have metabolic properties that naturally create traces of alcohol. This is a natural process of fermented foods. Many of these foods also produce vinegars such as lactic acid which is beneficial to the body. Many types of microflora that inhabit our gut live in these cultured foods. By keeping cultured food at home, we can provide a boost to our bodies' digestive system and reduce the strain on the body from eating processed foods.

Lacto-Fermented Vegetables

Lacto-fermented vegetables are a great source of beneficial microflora. In old times, families would store their harvested vegetables with salt in stoneware crocks in a root cellar. Over the winter, these vegetables would slowly pickle and ferment, becoming tart and acidic. Lacto-fermentation comes from the lactobacillus microflora that are present in fresh vegetables. The vegetables are packed in salt water to inhibit the growth of bad bacteria until the benefical microflora can take over and transform the vegetables into pickles. As the beneficial microflora multiply, they release lactic acid that drops the pH of the vegetables, further preventing any bad bacteria from spoiling the food. Vegetables stored this way can be stored for a very long time, as long as they are kept relatively cold.

This process can be mimicked today by packing fresh vegetables in a glass jar and covering with a brine, or mixture of salt and water, and an air tight lid. For beginners, I highly recommend a starter solution such as Caldwell's or Body Ecology's culture that contains beneficial cultures to jump-start the lacto-fermentation process. It is important that the beneficial microflora get a head start in the fermentation process. A correctly made batch of lacto-fermented vegetables will smell clean, tart, and will make you hungry. The vegetables must stay submersed in the brine culture liquid to prevent them from molding. Toss anything that is slimy or smells bad. Glass canning jars can be used, or special air lock lids can be purchased online from several companies specializing in lacto-fermented vegetables. It is also good to know that the liquid from a successful batch of vegetables can be used to boost the microflora of the next batch. I had a jar of lacto-fermented garlic in the back of my fridge for two years. I would often use a ¼ cup of liquid from this garlic to start the next batch of salsa. The liquid had a strong garlic flavor, of course, but that's fine in salsa.

Lacto-Fermented Salsa

One of the first lacto-fermented vegetables we made at home was homemade salsa. This was an obvious first choice because our family was already eating salsa and chips regularly. Lacto-fermented salsa tastes the same as homemade salsa, but it also has the added benefit of lactic acid and beneficial microflora.

4 fresh tomatoes
1 onion, diced
4 cloves garlic
1 tbsp. dried cilantro or 2 tbsp. fresh cilantro chopped
1 tbsp. salt
1 tbsp. lemon juice
Optional, thinly sliced jalapeno pepper to taste
*1 packet of lacto-fermentation starter culture (such as Caldwell's), or 2-3 tbsp. of yogurt whey, raw milk whey, or juice from a previous batch of lacto-fermented vegetables.

Dice vegetables and place in mixing bowl (if slicing hot peppers, be sure not to touch the peppers with your hands – wear gloves). Add salt and lemon juice and stir thoroughly. Mix 1 cup of water and starter culture, if using, and stir thoroughly into vegetables. Pack into quart size glass canning jar. Vegetables should come up to the neck of the jar, but not within about an inch of the top of the jar. Use remaining liquid to fill glass jar to within ¼" of the top, adding more water if necessary. Close lid tightly or add air lock at this time. Vegetables that didn't fit into the jar can be eaten anytime. Set at room temperature for 1-2 days then open and check for signs of fermentation. If using glass canning jars with metal lids, you may need to burp the jars by opening them slightly to let any air pressure escape.

You may see small bubbles forming in the liquid of the jar. This is good, showing that the fermentation is taking place. Warmer climates may need only 1 day to 12 hours for fermentation to take place. Move jar to refrigerator and enjoy.

Lacto-Fermented Bell Peppers

This is another great choice for families new to lacto-fermented foods. It's easy to take a chunk of bell pepper out of the jar in the fridge, dice, and add to creamy dips, salads, homemade pimento cheese, etc. As long as the food is not going to be cooked, you will keep all of the beneficial microflora from the lacto-fermentation in your creamy dip or salad.

The process is similar to the process of making salsa above, only it is necessary to remove the skins from the bell peppers first. Place 3-4 large bell peppers on a lightly oiled baking dish and bake at 400 for about 15 minutes, then turn over, and bake for another 10 minutes until skins shrivel. Allow peppers to cool enough to peel, then remove skins. Slice into quarters and place in mixing bowl. Add 1 tbsp. salt and 1 tbsp. lemon juice, 1 cup of water and starter culture if using. Mix thoroughly and pack into a quart size canning jar. Peppers should come up to the neck of the jar, but not within about an inch of the top of the jar. Use remaining liquid to fill glass jar to within ¼" of the top. Add more water if necessary. Set at room temperature for 1-2 days then open and check for signs of fermentation. If using glass canning jars with metal lids, you may need to burp the jars by opening them slightly to let any air pressure escape.

You may see small bubbles forming in the liquid of the jar. This is good, showing that the fermentation is taking place. A correctly made batch of lacto-fermented vegetables will smell clean, tart, and will make you hungry. Always toss any product that smells bad or is slimy. Move jar to refrigerator. Enjoy!

Lacto-Fermented Garlic

Another easy lacto-fermented vegetable that can be added to creamy dips, salsas, or just about anywhere where fresh garlic is called for. This also keeps in the refrigerator for a long time. It's easy to grab a clove of garlic out of the jar in the fridge and add to recipes. As long as the food is not going to be cooked, you will keep all of the beneficial microflora from the lacto-fermentation in your creamy dip or salad. Do not be alarmed if several of the cloves of garlic turn slightly blue or green in the fridge over time. This is normal and often happens to lacto-fermented garlic.

Peel fresh cloves of garlic. In a separate bowl, mix 1 tbsp. salt, 1 tbsp. lemon juice, 1 cup water and starter culture. Combine peeled garlic and liquid starter in a bowl and mix thoroughly. Pack garlic into a pint or quart size jar, depending on the number of fresh garlic cloves, to the neck of the jar, or within 1" of the top of the jar. Cover with liquid to within ¼" of the top of the jar. Close lid tightly or add air lock. Sit at room temperature for 1-2 days. Open and check for signs of fermentation. Then move to refrigerator for storage. Use as needed in recipes calling for fresh garlic, adding a small amount of water to keep garlic submersed in the liquid.

Water Kefir or "Homemade Soda"

Commercial sodas are detrimental to our health. What most people don't know is that there is a far healthier and tasty option! Water kefir is a homemade fizzy, bubbly drink made from water, sugar and fruit juice. Almost any type of fruit juice can be used making an endless variety of combinations a possibility. It makes a fantastic drink that kids love and an easy introduction to living foods for adults.

Water kefir grains are a symbiotic colony of beneficial yeasts and probiotic bacteria. They look like little grains of rice or gelatin. They live in a jar of mixed sugar water and in return, release air and lactic acid into the liquid. After sitting at room temperature for 2-3 days, this liquid is poured off, straining the kefir grains and keeping them for the next use. The kefir liquid that has been poured off can be added to about a half cup of any type of fruit juice, then bottled into locking, flip-top bottles. The kefir digests some of the sugar in the juice, in return releasing more lactic acid and air, naturally carbonating the kefir and juice.

After 12-24 hours, these bottles are put in the refrigerator. The result is a bubbly, fizzy drink that is both tasty and full of probiotics. Some examples of fruit juices that can be used are strawberry, blackberry, blueberry, orange, lemon and mint, pineapple and ginger, apple and cinnamon, and grape juice. Using locking, flip-top bottles for the second fermentation helps to really build up carbonation.

Process: We keep our kefir grains in a glass half gallon jar with a plastic air lock lid. We bought our airlock lid from Perfect Pickler. This is optional; some people just keep a simple cotton cloth with a rubber band over the top of their kefir grains. A plastic fine mesh strainer is needed to strain the kefir grains and pour off the liquid. Those are available online from Cultures for Health. A reusable coffee filter will also work. The kefir grains feed best on raw sugar, or pure evaporated cane juice. It has enough minerals to support the kefir grains. White sugar can be used, but the kefir grains will need a mineral boost from a spoonful of molasses or a few drops of Concentrace brand mineral drops on occasion; perhaps once a month. When you first purchase your kefir grains, they may be dehydrated in the packaging. Follow the instructions to rehydrate them. You may need to discard the first 1-3 batches of kefir water until the community of yeasts and bacteria balances and is thriving.

Gather 2-3 clean, flip-top bottles (a half gallon glass jar with an air tight lid will also work). Place a small funnel in the first bottle. Add the selected amount of fruit juice to each empty bottle. Then place the plastic strainer in the funnel. Pour the liquid water kefir into each bottle until half an inch from the top of the bottle. As the kefir grains collect in the strainer, you may need to dump them into a cereal bowl if you have too many to fit in the strainer. Finish filling the other bottles with kefir water. Close and lock the flip-top lids. Set these bottles aside for 12-24 hours, then place in the fridge. They will be ready to drink after about 12 hours but will still be mildly sweet. Longer time at room temperature builds up carbonation and reduces sugar content.

In a separate bowl, mix 1/4 cup of brown sugar with non-chlorinated water. Stir until dissolved. Add this sugar water to the original half gallon jar that was holding the kefir grains. Add the kefir grains. Fill the jar with room temperature, non-chlorinated water to within an inch of the top of the jar. Put the lid or cotton cloth back on the jar. Now the kefir grains are ready to sit happily in a dark location and bubble and ferment for 2-3 days. Colder locations may take a little longer to ferment.

If the colony of yeast and bacteria begins to get off balance, try some of these troubleshooting tips. If a "yeast" smell begins to develop, add a tablespoon of lemon juice to the kefir grains to lower the pH. This helps reduce the yeast population, allowing the beneficial bacteria population to strengthen. Also try rinsing the kefir grains under running water, then placing in a new, clean glass jar.

Note: Too much minerals, especially adding too much molasses or Concentrace mineral drops, can cause the kefir grains to suffer. Use only brown sugar until the grains begin to plump up and multiply again.

Composition: What exactly is water kefir? Water kefir consists of a symbiotic community of bacteria and yeast. The make-up of water kefir varies greatly depending on the culturing location and temperature. There are four women in my family maintaining water kefir grains, and each has a slightly different flavor. Water kefir has its own nuances. However, Cultures for Health lists some commonly found strains of bacteria and yeast in water kefir grains on their website. The strains listed may include many subspecies and variants:

Bacteria

Species Lactobacillus

L. brevis
L. casei
L. hilgardii
L. hordei
L. nagelii

Species Leuconostoc

L. citreum
L. mesenteroides

Species Acetobacter

A. fabarum
A. orientalis

Species Streptococcus

S. lactis

Yeasts

Hanseniaospora valbyensis
Saccharomyces cerevisiae
Zygotorulaspora florentina

*www.culturesforhealth.com/learn/water+kefir/composition-of-water-kefir-grains-bacteria-and-yeasts/. For general information purposes only.

Recipes: Pure water kefir does not have much flavor on its own. The second bottling and fermentation stage is what gives homemade soda it's great flavor and fizziness. Here are some examples of juices and flavor combinations to add to the water kefir for the second fermentation cycle. Keep in mind that bitter juices, such as lemon and cranberry, will need to have a little sugar added to sweeten the juice. Because the juice is added to the second fermentation, you can experiment all you want without effecting the kefir grains. Adjust these juices to suit your taste:

1/2 cup grape juice
1/2 cup blackberry juice
1 cup apple juice (apple juice has a milder flavor, so a little more juice helps strengthen the flavor), optional: a small cinnamon stick or a pinch of cinnamon
1/2 cup blueberry juice
1/2 cup pineapple juice with a thin slice of fresh ginger or coconut
1/2 cup orange juice
1 cup watermelon juice

Milk Kefir

This is another great product for culturing probiotics. Milk kefir tastes like a thin, creamy yogurt and can be bought at a grocery store or made at home. Milk kefir grains look like little grains of rice, similar to water kefir grains, except they are white. These grains look like they are made from gelatin and live in a small jar of milk kept in the fridge. Milk kefir is simple to make. It can be enjoyed plain, sweetened and flavored, or used in recipes such as Ranch dressing in the "Herbs" section of this book.

Process: Milk kefir is created by adding milk to milk kefir grains and yields a probiotic rich drink. Culture the grains in a quart jar filled with milk at room temperature. Cover jar with a cloth secured with a rubber band. Culture until the milk has slightly thickened, about 24 hours or less for warmer climates. After culturing is complete, strain the milk kefir grains out of the kefir through a plastic strainer. Add the kefir grains to a new jar of milk. The finished kefir can be flavored then stored in the fridge.

Kefir grains can be stored in the fridge for a few days to slow down fermentation. To culture refrigerated kefir grains, remove from fridge and allow to warm to room temperature. Strain and add kefir grains to new jar of milk, allowing to culture for 24 hours. Strain and move kefir grains to new jar of milk and place in the fridge.

Composition: Milk kefir consists of a symbiotic community of bacteria and yeast. The make-up of milk kefir varies greatly depending on the culturing location and temperature. Cultures for Health lists some commonly found strains of bacteria and yeast in milk kefir grains on their website. The strains listed may include many subspecies and variants. The cultures in milk kefir feed off of the lactose (milk sugar) and create a creamy, yogurt-like drink. The following list is bacteria and yeast found in different regions from 2 scientific studies. This list is for general information purposes only.

Bacteria

Lactobacillus acidophilus
Lactobacillus brevis
Lactobacillus casei
Lactobacillus delbrueckii subsp. bulgaricus
Lactobacillus delbrueckii subsp. delbrueckii
Lactobacillus delbrueckii subsp. lactis
Lactobacillus helveticus
Lactobacillus kefiranofaciens subsp. kefiranofaciens
Lactobacillus kefiri
Lactobacillus paracasei subsp. paracasei
Lactobacillus plantarum
Lactobacillus rhamnosus
Lactobacillus sake
Lactococcus lactis subsp. cremoris
Lactococcus lactis subsp. lactis
Lactococcus lactis
Leuconostoc mesenteroides subsp. cremoris
Leuconostoc mesenteroides subsp. dextranicum
Leuconostoc mesenteroides subps. mesenteroides
Pseudomonas
Pseudomonas fluorescens
Pseudomonas putida
Streptococcus thermophilus

Yeasts

Candida humilis
Kazachstania unispora
Kazachstania exigua
Kluyveromyces siamensis
Kluyveromyces lactis
Kluyveromyces marxianus

Saccharomyces cerevisiae
Saccharomyces martiniae
Saccharomyces unisporus

*www.culturesforhealth.com/learn/milk-kefir/milk-kefir-grains-composition-bacteria-yeasts/. For general information purposes only.

Recipes: Once the milk kefir is made and strained from the kefir grains, the milk kefir can be flavored any number of ways. Honey, vanilla, and fresh fruit can be used to create many flavor varieties. Have fun flavoring your kefir and see what kinds of combinations your family enjoys.

Kombucha

Kombucha (kum-BOOCH-a) is a fizzy, effervescent drink that can be made at home or purchased in grocery stores. It is made from tea and can be sweetened with fruit or juices. It is similar to water kefir, but stronger in flavor with a pronounced "vinegary" taste. In 2010, some bottled kombucha on shelves was found to contain up to 2.5% alcohol. Commercially made kombucha is now regulated by the government and manufacturers have changed some of their processes to reduce the alcohol content. Be sure to read labels and know what you and your family are consuming. The traditional process for making kombucha at home naturally reduces the alcohol content to trace levels. Making kombucha at home is fairly simple.

Process: You will first need to purchase a kombucha scoby from a health food store or an online store that sells starter cultures, such as Cultures for Health. Follow the instructions to activate your scoby. Brew one quart of hot tea and add ¼ cup of sugar. Stir to dissolve the sugar and allow the tea to steep for 10 minutes. Remove the teabag and cool to room temperature. Remove the scoby from your batch of kombucha and set aside on a clean plate. Pour off kombucha into a one quart jar or air-lock bottles, reserving ½ cup of kombucha for the next batch. Optional, to add more carbonation, add ½ cup of fruit juice for a second fermentation. Allow to set at room temperature for 24 hours and then place in the fridge. Once cooled, it is ready to drink.

Add ½ cup of kombucha from the previous batch to the newly made sweet tea. Replace the scoby to the new tea. Place a cloth filter over the top of the jar using a rubber band to secure the cloth. Allow the culture to sit undisturbed at room temperature, out of direct sunlight, 7-30 days or to taste. Dab the cloth with vinegar to help prevent mold growth.

Composition: The cultures in kombucha feed off of the sugar in sweetened tea. The culture is a symbiotic colony of bacteria and yeast that give the drink its flavor and carbonated fizz. Every culture of kombucha differs depending on the region and temperature where it's grown. Cultures for Health lists some strains that have been recorded in studies.

Acetobacter xylinoides
Acetobacter ketogenum
Saccharomycodes ludwigii
Saccharomycodes apiculatus
Schizosaccharomyces pombe
Zygosaccharomyes
Saccharomyces cerevisiae
Brettanomyces
Lactobacillus
Pediococcus
Gluconacetobacter kombuchae
Zygosaccharomyces kombuchaensis

*For general information purposes only. For more information, visit www.culturesforhealth.com.

Yogurt

Another easy option for getting probiotics into your diet is yogurt. Whole milk yogurt is best, especially any from pasture-raised cows. Commercially made yogurt will be pasteurized, which eliminates the live cultures naturally found in the milk. However, commercial companies will then add several strains of culture to ferment the milk into yogurt. Read the ingredients list on the back of the carton, which should list the strains of culture that have been added. Pick a yogurt that has at least several strains of live cultures.

Living foods on the road

Always pack a cooler with enough living foods to keep your gut in check as you indulge in vacation foods. This can be accomplished by packing or buying from grocers: water kefir, milk kefir, yogurts, lacto-fermented salsa, frozen raw milk, or kombucha. When traveling, local farmer's markets can also be a great source for fresh, local foods and homemade foods.

SALT AND MINERALS

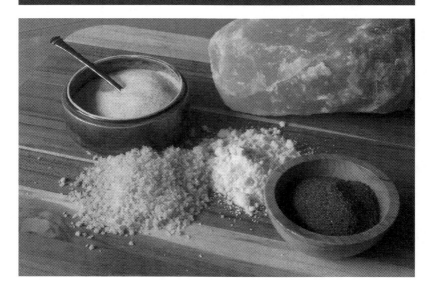

Salt has been indispensable for thousands of years. Our planet has an abundance of salty ocean water and numerous dried salt flats. Natural sea salt can be found in two forms: dehydrated salt water (sea salt) and salt mined from ancient salt beds such as the ones found near Salt Lake City, Utah and the Dead Sea. Mined salt can be white or pinkish in color, such as pink crystal salt. Evaporated seawater turns into light grey salt crystals when dried in the sun, such as Celtic salt. It contains about 14 percent macro-minerals, especially magnesium, and about 80 trace minerals, including iodine.[35] This magnesium is important in today's high-sugar diets (to metabolize sugar, the body has to use up large amounts of minerals and enzymes, around 56 molecules of magnesium for every one molecule of sugar).[36] Salt is also essential for digestion and activates enzymes in the intestines.[37] Salt is a great addition to food, and is essential for bone broths.

Bone broths contain many dissolved minerals, such as calcium, iodine, magnesium, potassium, and various trace minerals. Other great sources for minerals are pastured beef liver, which contains all of the fat-soluble vitamins A, D, E and K, all of the B vitamins in abundance (particularly vitamin B12), one of the best sources of natural folate, a highly usable form of iron and trace elements such as copper, zinc, and chromium.[38]

Epsom salts

Epsom salts are another great source for magnesium. Bath water and foot soaks are perfect because magnesium is better absorbed through the skin. A relaxing foot soak can be made by adding ¼ - 1/3 cup Epsom salts to warm water.

Authentic Fish sauce (the original soy sauce)

The only ingredients in an authentic fish sauce are fish and salt. To make this sauce, small fish such as anchovies are packed with salt and slowly fermented over time. This salty, mineral-rich sauce is difficult to find in most grocery stores but can be readily found in Asian or Indian grocery stores. It can also be purchased online.

Cast iron frying pans

Cast iron frying pans naturally add iron to foods cooked in them. They also absorb the flavors of the foods cooked in them and retain heat very well. They are one of my favorite additions to the kitchen. Avoid cooking acidic foods, like tomato sauces or citrus juices, because it can strip the seasoning from the pans causing food to stick.

Why Break Up With Salt?

Recently, there has been much energy spent making people aware of the dangers of salt in the diet. These discussions do not address the refining of salt and the havoc that refined salt has on the body.[39] Table salt has been refined and most of the naturally-occurring minerals are lost as a result. Anti-caking agents are then added to make the salt flow freely. This processing reduces the nutritional quality of the salt. Dr. Natasha Campbell-McBride writes, "Natural crystal salt and whole sea salt contain all of the minerals and trace elements, which the human body is made of. In this natural state is not only good for us, but essential. Because the industry requires pure sodium chloride, all the other elements and minerals get removed from the natural salt. We consume it under the name of "table salt" and of course all our processed foods contain plenty of it. This kind of salt comes into the body like a villain, upsetting our homeostasis on the most basic level. Our bodies have been designed to receive sodium chloride in combination with all

---

the other minerals and trace elements which a natural salt would provide. Pure sodium chloride draws water to itself and causes water retention with many consequences, such as high blood pressure, tissue oedema and poor circulation. As the body tries to deal with the excess of sodium chloride, various harmful acids and gall bladder and kidney stones are formed. As sodium in the body works in a team with many other minerals and trace elements (potassium, calcium, magnesium, copper, zinc, manganese, etc.), the levels of those substances get out of normal balance. The harmful results of table salt consumption can be numerous and very serious. That is why most medical practitioners, including the mainstream doctors, tell us not to consume table salt."

It is important to remember that sea salt is an important source of minerals and can be used in the diet. These campaigns against salt do not discuss that there is a healthy alternative. People then come to the wrong conclusion that *all* salt is bad. Sea salt is a vital part of a healthy diet.

NATURAL SUGARS

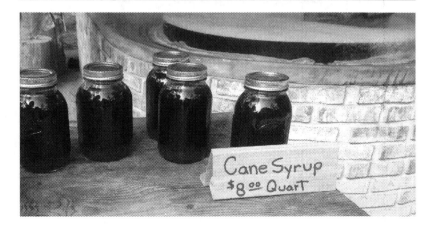

Where can we add sugar? In meat rubs and cures with salt and smoke! And rich desserts with cream and eggs. *Not* in drinks that are sipped all day long. Honey can be used with tea for coughs and sore throat, but for the most part, sugar should be eaten with protein and fats found in meat and desserts containing rich cream or eggs.

God has put natural barriers on the foods we should eat in small quantities. By His design, they are harder to come by in nature than meat and vegetables. One of these foods is sugar. A close look at the way God designed our planet will reveal that sugar is labor intensive. It takes a lot of work to get a pound of sugar without modern day factories cranking out large amounts of sugar. If we could rewind about a hundred years ago, we would find that harvesting sugar was a community effort that required many people working together for one annual harvest season.

The traditional process of making sugar and syrup requires time and patience. Some popular forms of sugar are maple syrup and cane syrup, which are made from plant sap collected from maple trees or sugar cane. The plant sap is a mildly sweet and very watery liquid. The sugar water is boiled down and reduced until it becomes a thick syrup. Gallons upon gallons of this sweet water must be collected to end up with one gallon of syrup. Once the sugar or syrup was produced, it was shared amongst those families who had gathered to produce the syrup. It had to last until the next year's harvest season. There's a sugarcane farm just north of where we live that hosts an annual sugarcane festival. One of the gentlemen working there told me that cane syrup is produced there at a 10:1 ratio, meaning for every gallon of syrup, they must render 10 gallons of sugar cane sap. Maple syrup is produced at a 40:1 ratio.

I recommend using the most natural source of sugar you can find, be it honey, cane syrup, maple syrup, or raw sugar. Natural sugars are typically brown, have a rich and flavorful aroma, and are full of minerals.

Simple Jams
(Easily spooned onto toast, pancakes, oatmeal, yogurt.)

We love making homemade jams, but we don't add half as much sugar as most recipes call for. Instead, we start with high quality, ripe fruit. The benefit of making jams this way is that they taste really good! The down side of using less sugar is that you cannot can them in a boiling water bath for storage later. They must be stored in the fridge.

Buy the best quality fruit you can afford. Produce from the grocery store often is picked green and allowed to ripen while in transit. This type of fruit does not make good quality jams. Hunt for fresh fruit that is local, or at least sold as tree-ripened. Fruit that is jam-worthy should taste sweet and delicious when eaten fresh. Strawberries should taste sweet, not bitter. Peaches should be sweet and tender, not mealy. Under ripe fruit requires more sugar to offset any bitter flavors and will not have that naturally sweet, fruity flavor that you're looking for in a great jam. U-pick farms are often a great place to get fresh, tree-ripened fruit at affordable prices.

Blueberry Spice Jam

4 pints fresh blueberries
2 cups sugar
A sprinkle of cinnamon, to taste

This recipe is actually a very simple spiced blueberry conserve, or a soft jam. Add 4 pints blueberries into a large pot and begin heating on medium-low heat. Add sugar and cinnamon. Begin to gently mash the berries with a potato masher. Turn up to medium heat and bring to a boil. Boil for one minute and then remove from heat. Ladle into quart or pint size jars for fridge storage.

Strawberry Jam

2 quarts ripe, sweet strawberries
2 cups sugar

Add strawberries to a large pot and begin heating on medium-low heat. Add 2 cups sugar and begin to gently mash the berries with a potato masher. Turn up to medium heat and bring to a boil. Boil for one minute and then remove from heat. Ladle into quart or pint size jars for fridge storage.

Strawberry Vanilla Jam Variation: Add vanilla bean seeds from one vanilla bean pod. Add right after adding sugar.

Sugar Plums

Sugar plums are a fun treat to have around the holidays and a fun way to get your kids to eat dried fruit. To make sugar plums, start with one cup of fresh dates (about 10-15 dates). Fresh dates are tasty and help hold the dried fruit mixture together. Slice open dates and remove seeds (fresh dates are perfect, dried dates may be too firm to work properly). Place pitted dates in food processor. Add extracts, additional dried fruit if desired, and mix until thoroughly blended. Some sample flavor combinations are:

Fresh dates, dried cranberries, orange extract
Fresh dates, dried blueberries, dash of cinnamon, ground clove
Fresh dates, dried pineapple, dried coconut, orange extract
Taking one tablespoon at a time, mold into small balls no larger than 1" in diameter. Roll each ball in powdered sugar, course sugar (raw sugar), or dip in melted chocolate. Place each sugar plum in a mini muffin cup liner. Coarse brown sugar can be powdered by placing in a coffee grinder.

Simple pies and cobblers

Start with high quality, ripe fruit. Cook fruit in a frying pan, adding ½ - ¾ cup of sugar. The recipe below can be followed using almost any kind of fruit. For apple or blueberry pie, sprinkle fruit with 1/8 – ¼ teaspoon of cinnamon.

Peach Cobbler

Begin by slicing 4 very ripe, sweet peaches into slices about ½ to ¾ of an inch thick. Preheat oven to 350F. Melt about 1 tablespoon of butter in a frying pan, adding sliced peaches. Cook on medium heat until peaches are tender, about 5 minutes. Add ½ cup sugar and continue stirring until sugar has dissolved into juice from peaches. Optional: add a light sprinkle of nutmeg or clove to make a "spiced" peach filling. Remove from heat. Pour the cooked peaches into a glass pie dish.

Topping: With a fork, mix in a separate bowl 1 cup flour, ½ tsp. salt, 2 tbsp. sugar, 4 tbsp. softened butter.

Mash with fork until crumbly. The flour will begin to form into rough crumbles that stick together when pressed but fall apart and crumble when stirred. It should not be one lump of dough or look like dry flour. If too dry, add a little more softened butter. If too sticky and forming into dough, add more dry flour. Sprinkle the crumbles onto hot cooked sweetened peaches in the pie dish. Bake at 350 for about 10 minutes or until browned.

***See the section about eggs for dessert recipes that include eggs, such as Vanilla Pie, Banana Pie and Eggnog.

Romans 11:33-36

Oh, the depth of the riches of the wisdom and knowledge of God! How unsearchable his judgments, and his paths beyond tracing out! "Who has known the mind of the Lord? Or who has been his counselor?"

"Who has ever given to God, that God should repay him?"

For from him and through him and to him are all things.

To him be the glory forever! Amen!

Index

Endnotes

All scripture and footnotes are from the NIV Study Bible published by Zondervan, 2008.

1　Fulbright, Jeannie, and Brooke Ryan, M.D. *Exploring Creation with Human Anatomy and Physiology.* Anderson, IN: Apologia Educational Ministries, Inc., 2010. Page 233. Print.

2　Campbell-McBride, Dr. Natasha. *Gut and Psychology Syndrome.* Revised Ed. Cambridge: Medinform Publishing, 2012. Page 261. Print.

3　United States Department of Agriculture. "Dietary Guidelines for Americans 2015-2020." Web. 2017.

4　*Food, Inc.* An Alliance Film, 2008. DVD.

5　Kolata, Gina. "In Good Health? Thank Your 100 Trillion Bacteria." *Nytimes.com.* The New York Times. June 13th, 2012. Web. 2016.

6　"Labeling Opponents." *Just Label It.* Nov. 2012. Web. 2017.

7　Ford, Dana, and Lorenzo Ferrigno. "Vermont Governor Signs GMO Food Labeling into Law." *Cnn.com.* CNN, May 8th, 2014. Web.

8　Addady, Michal. "President Obama Signed this GMO Labeling Bill." *Fortune.com.* Fortune. July 31st, 2016. Web.

9　*Food, Inc.* An Alliance Film, 2008. DVD.

10　United States Supreme Court. *OSGATA Organic Seed Growers and Trade Association, et al. v. Monsanto.* Filed by Public Patent Foundation. U.S. Supreme Court. Jan. 13th, 2014.

11 Hershberger, Vernon. Home page. 2016. Trial referenced is *State of Wisconsin vs. Vernon Hershberger.* Trial occurred May 20th-May 24th in Baraboo, Wisconsin. Web.

12 Darlington, Andre. "Don't Say 'Raw Milk' at the Vernon Hershberger Trial." *Isthmus.com.* May 21st, 2013.

13 Campbell-McBride, Dr. Natasha. *Gut and Psychology Syndrome.* Revised Ed. Cambridge: Medinform Publishing, 2012. Page 54. Print.

14 United States Department of Agriculture, National Agriculture Library. *Report of the Commissioner of Agriculture for the Year 1862.* Thirty-Seventh Congress, Session II. Chapter 72: An Act to Establish a Department of Agriculture, p. 387 and 388. Web.

15 Unger, Merrill F. *The New Unger's Bible Dictionary.* Ed. R.K. Harrison. Moody Bible Institute of Chicago. Moody Publishers. 1988. Print.

16 Price, Dr. Weston A. *Nutrition and Physical Degeneration.* Lemon Grove, CA: Price-Pottenger Nutrition Foundation, 2008. Page 25, 34. Print.

17 Pottenger, Jr., Dr. Francis M. *Pottenger's Cats.* Lemon Grove, CA: Price-Pottenger Nutrition Foundation, 2012. Page 39. Print.

18 Kolata, Gina. "In Good Health? Thank Your 100 Trillion Bacteria." *Nytimes.com.* The New York Times. June 13th, 2012. Web. 2016.

19 Dahl, Wendy J., and Volker Mai. "Go with Your Gut: Understanding Microbiota and Prebiotics." *University of Florida IFAS Extension*, Publication #FSHN11-10. Florida, June, 2011. Web.

20 Kolata, Gina. "In Good Health? Thank Your 100 Trillion Bacteria." *Nytimes.com.* The New York Times. June 13th, 2012. Web. 2016.

21 Campbell-McBride, Dr. Natasha. *Gut and Psychology Syndrome.* Revised Ed. Cambridge: Medinform Publishing, 2012. Page 31. Print.

22 The Gardeners and Farmers of Terre Vivante. *Preserving Food Without Freezing or Canning.* Chelsea Green Publishing Company. Vermont, 1999. Centre Terre Vivante is an ecological research and education center located in Mens, Domaine de

Raud, a region of southeastern France. Reference taken from page xx, Introduction. Print.

23 Campbell-McBride, Dr. Natasha. *Gut and Psychology Syndrome.* Revised Ed. Cambridge: Medinform Publishing, 2012. Page 16. Print.

24 Fallon, Sally. *Nourishing Traditions.* New Trends Publishing. Washington, D.C., 1999. Page 57. Print.

25 Campbell-McBride, Dr. Natasha. *Gut and Psychology Syndrome.* Revised Ed. Cambridge: Medinform Publishing, 2012. Page 42. Print.

26 Campbell-McBride, Dr. Natasha. *Gut and Psychology Syndrome.* Revised Ed. Cambridge: Medinform Publishing, 2012. Print.

27 Fallon, Sally. *Nourishing Traditions.* New Trends Publishing. Washington D.C., 1999. Page 46. Print.

28 Campbell-McBride, Dr. Natasha. *Gut and Psychology Syndrome.* Revised Ed. Cambridge: Medinform Publishing, 2012. Page 132. Print.

29 Schmid, ND, Ron. *The Untold Story of Milk.* New Trends Publishing, Inc. Washington D.C., 2009. Page 175, 181. Print.

30 Campbell-McBride, Dr. Natasha. *Gut and Psychology Syndrome.* Revised Ed. Cambridge: Medinform Publishing, 2012. Page 132. Print.

31 Schmid, ND, Ron. *The Untold Story of Milk.* New Trends Publishing, Inc. Washington D.C., 2009. Page 175, 181. Print.

32 Becker, Sue. *The Essential Home-Ground Flour Book.* Robert Rose, Inc. Toronto, Ontario, Canada. 2016. Page 26, 30, 58. Print.

33 Reinhart, Peter. *The Bread Baker's Apprentice: Mastering the Art of Extraordinary Bread.* Ten Speed Press. Berkeley, California. 2001. Page 29. Print.

34 Becker, Sue. *The Essential Home-Ground Flour Book.* Robert Rose, Inc. Toronto, Ontario, Canada. 2016. Page 22. Print.

35 Fallon, Sally. *Nourishing Traditions.* New Trends Publishing. Washington, D.C., 1999. Page 49. Print.

36 Campbell-McBride, Dr. Natasha. *Gut and Psychology Syndrome.* Revised Ed. Cambridge: Medinform Publishing, 2012. Page 111, 112. Print.

37 Fallon, Sally. *Nourishing Traditions*. New Trends Publishing. Washington, D.C., 1999. Page 48. Print.

38 Fallon, Sally. *Nourishing Traditions*. New Trends Publishing. Washington, D.C., 1999. Page 41, 49, 116-118. Print.

39 Campbell-McBride, Dr. Natasha. *Gut and Psychology Syndrome*. Revised Ed. Cambridge: Medinform Publishing, 2012. Page 141. Print.

Printed in the United States
By Bookmasters